Pregnancy 911-
The Weight Is Over!

G. Douglas Wood, M.D.

DEDICATION

To My Wife- I'm glad we found each other.

CONTENTS

ACKNOWLEDGMENTS

I want to thank and give my appreciation to the best office staff- Amy, Bonnie, and Cristen for all their help and support in caring for our patients. I want to thank Gabriel Decker for his helpful edits. I want to thank Lee Colwell for his genuine interest, review, and encouragements. I want to thank Scott Stanwood, Lou DeCaprio and Kristina Spellman, aka the Bostonian trio, for their help, and shared passion on this project. I want to thank maternal fetal medicine specialists Richard H. Aubry, MD, MPH of Syracuse, New York and James Meserow, MD of Chicago, Illinois for their assistance and input. Thanks to my best friend Stephen Carleson for the motivation and encouragement. I have to thank my kids, in order of appearance: Lauren, Hunter, Lindsey, Hudson, Audrey, Erin, and Henry for the fun distractions and play time breaks from the writing. Lastly, I want to thank my wife for her help and encouragement along the way.

INTRODUCTION

Congratulations! If you're reading this book it's likely that you are pregnant, contemplating pregnancy, or you have recently delivered. Regardless of the circumstance, it's important that you have recognized the importance of nutrition. Nutrition has been little more than casual conversation in the health and medical fields, until recent years. Why should it? We live in the land of plenty. We have the largest supply of food in our history; yet we are starving. Our society is malnourished and starving for good and appropriate nutrition. I know this for a fact because I see it every day in my medical practice. Not only do I see it on a daily basis in my medical practice, but I have experienced it firsthand.

I spent my childhood, adolescent years, and the majority of my adulthood being skinny, not by choice, I ate everything all the time. I couldn't gain weight if I tried. Don't hate me, let me finish. As early adulthood progressed, I slowly obtained a normal weight for my height. I finally looked healthy and not so skinny. I was blessed with a fast metabolism, and I didn't have to change much to maintain my weight and appearance. However, over the past several years, I have walked down the road that waits for most of us. I noticed I crept up a few pounds. I shrugged it off and told myself not to worry, unless I gained another few pounds. Then, along with the next few months came the next few pounds. I told myself it was a fluke and the weight gain would stop. Again, I would not worry unless I went up another few pounds. Within a few more months, I was up a few more pounds and now a lot of my clothes were not fitting. I adopted a new philosophy of "fat and happy". I figured it was time for me to just be fat and happy.

Things were going good, and I was happy, but I could not see physically what was happening. I looked the same to myself. Then, it hit me like a ton of bricks when I was looking at pictures from a recent vacation. We were at a water park and I was standing next to my pregnant wife. I was looking at that picture and I saw my beautiful wife who was 3 weeks from delivering our last child, and me standing next to her. I thought, is that really me! If so, when was my estimated due date. I looked like I was starting my third trimester. What a look for someone who wasn't pregnant. I could not believe it, how did I get from lean trim 135 pounds to 175 pounds! I decided then and there to do something about it.

I already knew the science of metabolism; I just needed to apply it. I researched the current literature and read several books on weight loss and diets. I didn't realize how much confusion and misinformation was out there. I discovered how difficult it was to actually find nutritious food. I formulated a nutritional plan and my wife and I started it right after she delivered our youngest son. Our goal, was to get back to a normal healthy BMI and adopt a healthy nutritional lifestyle within 3 months. I focused our plan around increased lean protein and healthy sources of nutritional carbohydrates along with strength training exercises. All of which I will discuss in detail later in the book. We achieved our goal within three months. We felt better and had more energy than we have had in years. We won the battle! Even better, we got control back of our nutrition, health and weight. I cannot tell you enough, how good it feels to have a healthy control over your weight. It is a great feeling. An empowering feeling! People who have been there know exactly what I am talking about, and you will too! It's powerful!

I mentioned earlier, I frequently see malnutrition in my medical practice. I am an obstetrician and gynecologist with a large obstetrical practice. In fact, as of this writing I have managed and delivered over 6,200 pregnancies. During this time, I spent several years making observations and notes in my practice regarding nutrition during pregnancy. I also researched back and studied what my field has to offer in terms of nutrition for obstetrical patients. Modern obstetrics has greatly reduced the morbidity and mortality associated with direct factors affecting childbirth. However, there has been a slight rise in the maternal mortality ratio over the past several years, largely contributed to indirect factors. Indirect factors include preexisting health conditions which are exacerbated by pregnancy. Overweight and obese conditions further complicate these indirect factors and conditions. Unfortunately, modern obstetrics has not made great strides in assuring a healthy nutritional lifestyle for expecting mothers. It is not surprising, the medical field as a whole has done little to help treat, or find the cure for our current epidemic. Obstetricians generally follow and practice the techniques they were taught during their residency training. Unfortunately, most of these programs lack a formal curriculum in nutritional training.

The training and practices are influenced by the American Congress of Obstetricians and Gynecologists. The American Congress of Obstetricians and Gynecologists, also referred to as ACOG, makes recommendations and guidelines for various issues and practices in the field of obstetrics and gynecology. With respect to obstetrical nutrition, ACOG recommends a certain minimum caloric intake depending on the trimester of pregnancy. There are no specific recommendations of the source of the calories. ACOG also recommends weight gain based on a person's pre-pregnancy weight, "a one size fits all," recommended weight gain during the pregnancy. Just get those calories and gain that weight! It is not surprising with that recommendation and the food supply that surrounds us, that over two thirds of pregnant women are either overweight or obese. The amount of pregnancy complications that are increased and the number of overweight newborns as a result are equally shocking.

I see this going on and the results of it every day. One of the mother's most common concerns at the postpartum visit is how to get rid of all the pregnancy weight that she gained while pregnant. I am here to tell you, "The weight is over!" I can help you. I am here to help you make a difference. Over the years, I have put together a healthy nutritional program that not only works, but allows the unborn child to grow, and prevents the mother from gaining any unnecessary weight. In fact, the mother is close to her pre-pregnancy weight shortly after delivery.

Together, we can cast the stone into the lake of plenty and start a nutritional ripple across the country that will have a positive effect on expecting mothers and their unborn children. It is a healthy nutritional lifestyle that everyone in the family can follow. Hopefully, together we can stop the nutritional epidemic that plagues us for our future generations. As you read this book and follow along towards a healthier nutritional lifestyle, here are a few tips to keep in mind to help with your understanding and success:

1.   Quality is more important than quantity. Pregnancy is not a time for calorie deprivation and in fact there are minimum recommendations for the number of calories depending on the trimester of pregnancy. The importance is in the type of nutrient or nutrients that the calories come from, because that determines the impact on metabolism and body composition. Attention must be paid to the types of proteins and carbohydrates and the relative proportions to each other. There are desirable proteins and carbohydrates that have a positive effect on body composition, and there are undesirable proteins and carbohydrates that have a negative effect on body composition. Knowing the differences, make a difference.

2.   Make more than a baby, make muscle too. Strength training is a must. Making more muscle is more important and more beneficial than aerobics. Strength training is not the same as bodybuilding; it is completely different. Muscle is a major fat burner and is your best friend when it comes to improving body composition. Strength training not only gives you the same healthy heart benefits of aerobics; it helps you create a lean sculptured body that constantly burns fat. These results cannot be achieved with aerobics. Although strength training is highly recommended and will help you achieve results faster, it is not mandatory. A healthier nutritional lifestyle and a better body composition can be achieved by nutrition alone. Move out fat, muscle is moving in.

3.   Think differently about food. Every meal should not be about entertaining your taste buds to the maximum. Focus should be on the purpose of your food, which is to nourish your body. Thinking smart about food choices will give you both a healthy nutritional choice that is also tasty, without sacrificing body composition. Remember, you are what you eat.

4.   What's good for the goose is good for the gander. The same nutritional ideas about obtaining a healthy nutritional lifestyle work the same for him too. My wife and I both take a team approach to nutrition. Knowing you are working as part of the team, particularly with a loved one, helping to improve each other's health increases your motivation and success. Those of you who are expecting or who already have children have

even more reasons to succeed. His work is not "already done" he has much more to do! So, go get him and the two of you start a healthier nutritional lifestyle together.

I follow the same nutritional lifestyle I recommend in my book. Not only do I talk the talk, I walk the walk. I have found that taking what I have learned inside and outside the hospital, I can help countless others to become healthier. Hopefully I can instill a healthier nutritional lifestyle in generations to come. Motivated by the fact that two thirds of pregnant women are either overweight or obese, and my strong desire to help you and countless others, I have teamed up with others to start a campaign to improve the nutritional lifestyle of pregnant women in this country. I challenge you to be part of our 20/20 OB Challenge. The campaign aims to improve, and/or impact in a positive manner, at least 20% of the overweight or obese pregnant women by the year 2020. It is hoped by accomplishing this goal that a movement will be put in place that will reverse the trend towards obesity in pregnant women and thereby improving the health and outcomes of not only pregnancies, but perpetuate a healthy nutritional lifestyle in future generations. I challenge you to follow this book and make a difference!

In good health, Douglas Wood, MD.

1 OB NUTRITIONAL SYSTEMS

OB Nutritional Systems is a nutritional program I developed to allow pregnant women to adopt and maintain a healthy nutritional lifestyle. Good news, understanding nutrition and how it impacts your body's metabolism is more than half the battle. This philosophy applies whether you are thinking about becoming pregnant, currently pregnant, or recently delivered. This philosophy also applies if you are already fit and in shape, and want to continue to maintain your figure during and after pregnancy. Those of you who are overweight may have a net loss in weight during your pregnancy, subsequently reducing pregnancy associated risk factors. The rest of the challenge is being motivated enough to stay on and maintain a nutritional plan that will meet your goals.

More good news! One of the most motivated times in a woman's life is during pregnancy. The reason being, she is motivated by the safety and well-being of her unborn child. The well-being of her child is, without a doubt, influenced by her nutrition. The best way to keep your baby healthy is to keep yourself healthy. This motivation can help you succeed in your nutritional goals and hopefully continue long after the pregnancy into a healthy nutritional lifestyle.

OB Nutritional Systems will teach you how to eat in a way that will work with your metabolism. This program will help you understand which foods to eat. It will help you combine nutrition and fitness to help you achieve healthy weight goals during and after your pregnancy. This program is not just for people who are fit, or for people trying to avoid any excess weight gain during pregnancy. OB Nutritional Systems will help those who have had disastrous results from previous pregnancies and who have fought a lifelong battle with being either overweight or obese. OB Nutritional Systems is designed to help all those who have tried to diet and control weight after their pregnancy with countless attempts at counting calories, but still continue to grow fat and overweight.

OB Nutritional Systems is a healthy nutritional lifestyle based on reviewing numerous nutritional programs, ACOG nutritional recommendations, review of research literature, personal experiences, and on my work as an obstetrician and gynecologist. The study of metabolism has provided us with the knowledge and information to maintain a healthy nutritional lifestyle without starving, cutting calories, or using dangerous drugs. The information gained by understanding metabolism often explains why the majority of people fail to maintain a healthy nutritional lifestyle, which is nearly 90% of the time. Understanding metabolism explains why people who eat the least often weigh the most and why most calorie counting programs fail. There is little left to wonder why Americans are growing fatter every year, and why maintaining a healthy nutritional lifestyle has become a major struggle for most Americans including our children!

I am a doctor, father of seven, husband and an excellent observer of details. My specialty is obstetrics and gynecology. During medical school, specialty training, and in my professional practice, I have always had an interest in both physiology and biochemistry as it relates to metabolism. I have seen the effects of good and poor nutrition on several thousand pregnancies thus far in my career. I have seen firsthand how nutrition plays an important role in the pregnancies of my own children. My wife and I use the same information every day to maintain a healthy nutritional lifestyle and set good examples for our children to follow. We do our part in helping break the cycle of obesity in our family. The experience I have gained and the observations I have made during the management of countless pregnancies over the years is invaluable. The extensive review of the available research and literature pertaining to metabolism and nutrition is endless. Combining the experience and research has helped me help others reduce pregnancy risks associated with excess weight, and make the information available so that I can help countless others help themselves to a healthy nutritional lifestyle. This, in turn, reduces excess weight resulting in better pregnancy outcomes.

Every mother, and couple, want to have a healthy pregnancy without complications. They want a nice healthy newborn baby that will grow up healthy and strong. Pregnant women like to brag a little when they are doing well during their pregnancy, or when their delivery was smooth and easy. But, they also have a rewarding smile of relief when they are back in their skinny jeans right after delivery, or by the end of their six week postpartum period. Maintaining a healthy nutritional lifestyle during pregnancy can give you these results, and help give you a strong healthy body with good muscle tone. A strong healthy body will be less likely to develop pregnancy complications such as gestational diabetes, preeclampsia, birth trauma, and operative deliveries such as a cesarean section. A healthy postpartum body makes an easier recovery, and an easier transition into continuing a healthy nutritional lifestyle. A lifestyle is learned in which the body is less likely to develop obesity, heart disease, diabetes, and countless other diseases that run rampant through our aging and overweight society.

OB Nutritional Systems is divided into five phases. There is one phase for each of the three trimesters of pregnancy. Each trimester is recognized because of the increased fetal growth and increased nutritional requirements as the pregnancy progresses through each trimester. The phases also take in consideration the changing maternal shape and physical limits. Phase four takes in consideration not only the recovery period but nutritional requirements related to breast-feeding. Phase five considers adapting a continual healthy nutritional lifestyle after the completion of your pregnancy. Part five can also be considered as a preconception phase as well. The OB Nutritional Systems meal plan will provide all the necessary nutritional requirements for your pregnancy, will leave you satisfied, eating more than you could dream possible, and help reduce some of the nausea that is often associated with pregnancy.

The strength training regimen, designed with pregnancy in mind, is kept simple and brief without hours of exercise videos and other time-consuming routines. As you follow the OB Nutritional Systems meal plan and exercise regimen you will notice a positive change in your body composition and energy. Remember, body composition is the ratio of lean body mass to fat mass. You will replace fat as you build muscle, which will add shape and tone to your body. A body with good shape and tone from a healthy nutritional lifestyle will feel better and have more energy, despite the energy draining effects of pregnancy.

Phase one, the first trimester phase, provides the necessary nutrition for your pregnancy. This phase begins training you on how to eat correctly, what foods to eat, and which foods to avoid. In this phase, you will develop a consistent nutritional routine, as well as, a consistent exercise routine to convert into good habits.

Phase 2 and phase 3, the second and third trimester phases, are simply modified progressions of phase 1. There are slight modifications to ensure adequate coverage of the increased demands of the continuing and growing pregnancy. Also, the slight variations to the exercise regimen account for the growing pregnancy.

Phase 4, the postpartum phase, focuses on recovering and breast-feeding. The body gradually transitions into phase 5. Phase 5 is the ongoing phase to maintain a healthy nutritional lifestyle which continues to provide you with a slim, lean and healthy body for life.

During the 11 months, from conception through postpartum, you will have significantly transformed your metabolism which will keep you stronger, healthier, and happier than you have been in the past. You will transition your body from a pre-pregnancy state, through pregnancy, postpartum, and back again with minimal adverse impact. You will most likely be in better shape than you were pre-pregnancy.

2 A GROWING AMERICA

Americans are a growing society, but not in a good way. Approximately 68.5% of adult Americans are overweight or obese. This equals about two- thirds of the population. In children between the ages of two through five years old, one out of four are overweight or obese. One-third of the American school age children are overweight or obese. Almost 36% of American adults are obese and almost 17% of American children and teenagers are obese. Well over half of all groups are overweight. The prevalence of obesity in America has increased steadily in the last few decades of the 20th century. At the present, there appears to be a slowing, or leveling off, of the rate of increase. But, the prevalence of obesity continues to remain constant. I encourage you to go for walk and look around. The next time you're at the mall, movies, or out to eat take notice of the people around you. When you're outdoors at a park, swimming pool, or an outdoor event look at the people around you. Next time you're near a school or a playground take a good look at the children. We live in a nutritional nightmare! You are not dreaming, it's for real. The prevalence of obesity in pregnancy is equally shocking. Two-thirds of all pregnant women are either overweight or obese. One-third of all pregnant patients are considered obese. 8% of pregnant patients are considered to be extremely obese. Over one-half of all pregnant patients are considered to be overweight. You should find this shocking; I know I did.

The body mass index, or BMI, is the assessment of weight relative to height of an individual. It is a useful screening tool to indirectly measure the amount of body fat of a person. Overweight is defined by having a body mass index between 25 and 29.9. Grade 1 obesity is a body mass index between 30 and 34.9. Grade 2 obesity is a body mass index between 35 and 39.9. Grade 3 obesity is a body mass index of 40 or greater. As I just mentioned, 35% of Americans are overweight, 20% have grade 1 obesity, 9% have grade 2 obesity, and 6% have grade 3 obesity. Why is this important? Excess body weight has a strong correlation with excess morbidity and mortality. In fact, grade 2 and above obesity significantly increases the risk of death. People with excess body weight and obesity are at higher risk for hypertension, adverse lipid concentrations, and type II diabetes. All three of these conditions increase the risk of heart disease. Remember, heart disease is the number one killer of women. Heart disease kills more women than lung and breast cancer combined. Obesity also increases your risk of developing three serious metabolic disorders. The three disorders are: Syndrome X or metabolic syndrome, insulin resistance, and type II or adult onset diabetes. All of these disorders involve an abnormal amount of insulin.

Insulin is a hormone that regulates the body's metabolism of sugar and starches, as well as many other important jobs. Insulin has a critical role in the storage of fat, protein, and the manufacture of cholesterol. The starchy and sugary foods, that are widespread throughout our food supply, cause a sharp rise in blood sugar which causes a spike in blood insulin levels. A chronic increased level of insulin can cause multiple medical problems throughout the body. Syndrome X, or metabolic syndrome, is a triad of medical problems which includes increased levels of triglycerides, high blood pressure, and high levels of insulin such as that found in type II diabetes. There is evidence to suggest that maternal metabolism and nutrition appear to program the fetal metabolism. The Barker Hypothesis suggests that sub-optimal nutrition and metabolic conditions can program the fetus in the direction of the Metabolic Syndrome. This condition leading to eventual susceptibility to hypertension and diabetes when the fetus becomes an adult.

Insulin resistance occurs when the target cells of insulin become resistant to hormones affects because of chronically high levels of insulin. Insulin resistance often presents itself in women with absent or infrequent menstrual cycles. Testing for this condition is often overlooked when women present with complaints of infrequent, or absent, periods. I always include a glucose and insulin level as part of the work up for these women. It is surprising how frequently this condition is found in this group of women. It is often missed and overlooked because a person's random blood sugar is often in the normal range, typically in the high normal range. If the insulin is measured, it will be found to be elevated and the ratio of glucose to insulin will be abnormally low. Insulin resistance can have a major adverse impact on women's fertility. Type II or adult onset diabetes is a condition where the insulin works less efficiently on the target organs. This disease increases the risk of heart disease, kidney damage, and blindness.

Unfortunately, in the recent decades we have seen this adult onset disease occurring in children. Childhood obesity is one of the top health concerns today. This concern out ranks drug abuse and smoking among children. We're now seeing problems in children that we have not seen in the past. These problems include: hypertension, type II diabetes, and increased cholesterol. Childhood obesity also leads to low self-esteem and depression among children.

Over the past four decades we have seen a steady increase in obesity in America. What is happening? Have Americans become lazy? Has the technology caused us to decrease the amount of exercise in our routine? There have been several studies that have looked at the physical activity and exercise in America. Despite the major advances in technology, computers, and videogames, the average daily physical activity has remained relatively constant if not slightly increased. Therefore, it does not have any statistical significance in explaining an impact on obesity. Studies have also looked at the overall consumption of food in America and it too is remained relatively constant. However, there has been significant changes and modifications in our food supply. So why has this happened? Why have we suddenly over the past few decades, become an extremely overweight and obese society? There have been many theories and explanations given; some people say Americans gorge on food and have become lazy, so lazy and inactive that we don't burn off excess calories; some say fast food restaurants are to blame with their supersized meals adding to the gluttony; some say that kids spend too much time playing video games, on the computer, and watching television.

Other people are quick to blame the problem of obesity on the "so-called" fat gene. There is no doubt that chronic overeating and lack of exercise will result in excess weight. I am sure that overconsumption and an inactive lifestyle will explain some of the increases in obesity. And, there are people who definitely have a genetic disposition to being heavy. These problems have been present in our society in one form or another for centuries. Therefore, none of these explanations can account for the marked increase in obesity that has occurred in just the past few decades. If it were true, it would mean that sometime around 1980 everyone in America started sitting down gorging and stopped exercising all at once. Also in 1980, the fat gene got turned on. None of this makes sense in explaining such a rapid increase in overweight and obese Americans since 1980.

Americans are not consuming significantly more calories than they used to, nor are they more sedentary than in the past. Physical activity in Americans has remained relatively constant. If the obesity in America is not being caused by eating too much, laziness, or genetics, then what is the cause? Remember, obesity and poor body composition, go hand-in-hand. Obese people have too much body fat and too little muscle. People are not born that way. The problem is the modern diet. I and several other providers and professionals believe that the sustained rise in obesity, that we've seen over the past several decades, is because of major changes in the Western diet that occurred during the same time periods. It's not from eating too much food. It's from eating too much of the wrong food.

When will you say enough is enough? We are rapidly approaching having three quarters of all American adults and one half of all the children being seriously overweight or obese. For you to know what you can do to help reverse this trend you have to understand why the rate of obesity began to escalate after 1980. You need to understand the events that led up to this nutritional nightmare.

High fructose corn syrup was invented in the late 1950's and started being used significantly starting in the 1960's. As a result of the increased cost of sucrose (table sugar), high fructose corn syrup became the major sweetener of choice by manufacturers, and essentially replaced sucrose in most instances. Incidentally, from 1970 thru the 1990's there was a 25% increase in the amount of sugar used in America. Wheat used to be a health food until in the mid-70s. The plant was reengineered. The once 4.5 feet tall wheat plant was modified to yield an 18 inch high-yielding plant. Unfortunately, the new wheat protein causes us to over eat. The wheat protein actually stimulates appetite. This modified wheat protein along with sucrose and high fructose corn syrup give individuals a euphoric feeling when consumed. They also cause a significant response in insulin which signals the body to remove sugar from your blood to your tissues. With high insulin levels, over time more and more sugar gets stored as fat. The increasing drop of sugar causes a loss of the euphoric feeling; therefor, a craving for more sugar and increasing appetite happens. It is a self-perpetuating problem.

Because products made with high fructose corn syrup as a preservative can be produced cheaper, they are more likely to show up on the grocery shelves, crowding out healthier foods. You don't have to take my word for it, just go to the grocery store. Go to the aisles and start looking at the ingredients on the product labels. You will find it difficult to find a product without high fructose corn syrup, sugar, or wheat listed in the first five ingredients. We are paying to be poisoned with these foods. We can change things. By making changes in our food selections that reflect a healthier nutritional lifestyle, we can then demand healthier foods, and stores will start stocking healthier foods at the expense of less healthier ones.

Another reason people have become overweight, or obese, is the lack of protein in their diets. Unfortunately, it has been crowded out on our plates by highly processed and refined foods. Primarily, starchy carbohydrates have taken over our food choices. Carbohydrates have not only taken over, but they have been reinforced by fast foods with high fat content. In just a few short decades protein has been pushed down from the primary nutrient source in our diets to being just an extra in the crowd. The modern diet obtains, on average, between 12 and 15% of the daily calories from protein. This may be enough to survive on but not nearly enough to thrive on. When protein is used as the primary nutrient in our diet, it helps prevent fat storage. Protein is used by the body to build muscle, repair and replace injured tissue, and can be used as an energy source. Protein cannot be used to make or store fat. Most carbohydrates, on the other hand, can readily be converted to fat storage. As part of a healthier nutritional lifestyle, protein must be reintroduced as the major nutrient in our diet.

The common link is nutrient partitioning. Nutrients can be either positive partitioning agents or negative partitioning agents. To avoid storing fat and build lean muscle mass, there must be positive partitioning nutrients to favor the fat burning, muscle building pathway. Consuming negative partitioning nutrients will cause you to be stuck in a fat storing pathway. The overall composition of food and nutrients, in the food we eat, determines which pathway is switched on. Unfortunately, over the past several decades, our food supply has become filled with foods and additives that are negative partitioning agents. Since 1980, negative partitioning agents have, all but, crowded out positive partitioning agents. As a result, people are getting fatter with each passing year. Sadly, some of these foods are being passed on to the American public as health foods. I believe, as well as many others, that public enemy number one is high fructose corn syrup. It is a food additive in the majority of foods we eat, and it is a particularly potent negative partitioning agent. It is felt to be responsible for the marked rise in obesity that started in the 1980s.

What about calories, don't they count? Doesn't eating too many calories make you fat? Cutting calories will make you slim, right? Calorie theorists and manufacturers, that rely on high fructose corn syrup, want you to think that way. Studies have shown that the human metabolism is far more complicated. Calorie intake by itself does not determine body composition. It is not about quantity; it is about quality. There are plenty of examples of people who eat low calories but still have a high amount of body fat. Weight they lose is from muscle as well as fat. Loss of muscle results in poor body composition and a subsequent breakdown in metabolism. There are plenty of examples, bodybuilders are an excellent example, of people who eat many more calories and become muscular and trim. This occurs because of nutrient partitioning. Nutrient partitioning keeps calories in check. The medical field is finally starting to recognize this phenomenon.

3 WHAT WE EAT MATTERS

People in this country have become increasingly overweight, or obese for the past four decades. For a long time, nutritionists, physicians, and researchers generally thought that metabolism works the same way regardless who we are or what we eat. The calorie equation had to balance. The number of calories we consumed would equal the amount of calories needed for energy; plus, the excess stored as fat. If there was a deficit it would have to equal a negative value; a negative value would equal weight loss. Therefore, those individuals who consume too many calories would store too much fat, and get fat. Individuals that ate too few calories would lose weight and become thin. Those concepts were more concerned about the quantity of food you ate instead of the quality of the food you ate. When I refer to quality of food, I am referring to the "nutritional" quality of the food. The nutritional quality determines how the food will interact with your metabolism and determines whether you will burn or store fat. Cutting calories, especially to a level well below a person's basal metabolic requirement, will definitely cause a loss in weight. But, the real question is what type of weight is lost; is the weight loss from fat, muscle, or water? It is likely a significant amount of all three.

With a very restricted caloric intake, fat is definitely consumed; but, under certain conditions there is a significant development of ketosis which results in a significantly equal loss of water to allow the body to flush the ketones through the kidneys and out through the urine. These diets are typically known as ketogenic diets. Ketosis occurs with a low calorie and low carbohydrate diet. This is characteristic of high protein low carbohydrate diets. Additionally, if inadequate protein is consumed on these diets, then there is a significant loss of muscle mass as well. Remember, muscle is a powerful fat burner. With the loss of muscle goes the loss of fat burning ability. With these types of diets people lose weight but at a high cost of losing muscle and water. This results in poor body composition and a "wasted look." Not to mention, people on these diets feel miserable and tired. Another phenomenon also occurs on low calorie diets. The metabolism slows in response, and further fat burning capacity is reduced. The body senses a starvation phase and slowly starts to shut or slow things down as much as possible in order to survive. There is no advantage for an organism to starve itself, only to defend itself from starving.

Also, there is no evolutionary or competitive advantage to starving. So, strictly and solely cutting calories is only part of the picture. Definitely not a method that would result in a healthy nutritional lifestyle in the long run.

The growing majority of nutritionists, scientists, and physicians, myself included, disagree with this idea of the calorie equation approach to nutrition. To understand weight management, you must understand and know about metabolism. Our body first breaks down food that we eat so that it can be absorbed. Then, these absorbed nutrients and particles are used by the body in various ways. This process is called metabolism. There is another metabolic factor called nutrient partitioning. This factor affects how our bodies handle our food and can either work for us or against us. When nutrients are broken down, they can be used for either energy or they can be stored. When nutrients are used for energy, they are burned off and consumed. Nutrients that are not used for energy are stored. They are stored either as fat deposits or in the form of lean muscle mass. The type of nutrient being metabolized has a significant impact on the type of storage. People have a metabolic tendency that they are born with and inherited genetically. This tendency can either store or burn fat. Everyone seems to know those few individuals that can eat any and everything and never gain weight. That person has the metabolic tendency to burn fat and store muscle; he/she is considered to be quite lucky.

The other two thirds of the population has the metabolic tendency to burn muscle and store fat. The reason there are many more people with a metabolic tendency to store fat is not because of chance. It happened because it was advantageous for our ancestors long ago and continued to be advantageous until a drastic change in food supply occurred in the last half of the 20th century. At one time food was scarce and starvation was a very real threat. Our ancestors, who had a metabolic tendency to store fat, were better able to survive. In today's society, food is plentiful and having a metabolic tendency to store fat is no longer beneficial, especially given the type of high carbohydrate and processed food supply that we have today. Thus, nutrient partitioning, coupled with the wrong type of nutrient being presented, is the culprit which leads us to store fat and results in the obesity.

Nutrient partitioning can be thought of as a metabolic fork in the road with two pathways. One pathway, we will call "A," and the other, we will call "B". As nutrients are consumed and used they can be directed into one of the two pathways depending on the type of nutrient presented at the metabolic fork. Directing nutrients to pathway A, our body converts the nutrients into muscle or lean body mass. This is the pathway we prefer to help us look fit and trim. Directing nutrients to pathway B, our body converts the nutrients into fat which becomes stored. We want to avoid this pathway in order to prevent unhealthy weight gain. Those individuals with a metabolic tendency to store fat have a tendency to direct nutrients to pathway B. Unfortunately, some of the foods we eat further favor directing the consumed nutrients to pathway B. A result of this is that too many nutrients are directed and stored as fat. Some of the most common ingredients in the food supply today are the worst offenders and favor our metabolic pathway B. The diet we consume today is filled with foods and additives that favor pathway B and shunt too many nutrients into fat storage. These foods and additives are called negative partitioning agents.

To further the problem, we have reduced the intake, and in some cases, eliminated the intake of the types of foods that favor pathway A. Foods that favor pathway A are called positive partitioning agents. When we consume nutrients we can take in either positive or negative partitioning agents. The goal of a healthy nutritional lifestyle is to maximize the intake of positive partitioning agents while minimizing or avoiding negative partitioning agents.

The primary purpose of OB Nutritional Systems is to use nutrient partitioning to an advantage. The importance is in the quality of the food that you eat and not the quantity. Focus on nutrient partitioning and not calorie counting. If you are able to eat a diet filled with foods that are positive partitioning agents, then you are able to eat as much as you want without regard to calories and not get fat. If you eat a diet filled with foods that are negative partitioning agents, then regardless of how much, or how little, you eat you will still become fat.

When you are in fat storage mode, or favoring pathway B, it's difficult to feel good. You gain excessive weight which is stored as body fat. Eventually, this results in you not only looking and feeling fat, but feeling bad about the way you look. Not to mention the increased health risks for yourself and your pregnancy. The excess body fat is what makes your body have to work harder, and fat stored in certain locations can lead to diseases of various organs such as heart disease. In pregnancy, it results in increased risk of hypertension, preeclampsia, and other metabolic disorders such as gestational diabetes. Excessive deposits of body fat in the pelvic region can increase the difficulty of delivery and can result in dystocia which disrupts the progress of labor and can result in a cesarean section.

Diet, exercise, and drugs are not the answer. You have to use healthy nutrition and an exercise regimen that turns away from pathway B (fat storing pathway) and turns in the direction of pathway A (fat burning pathway). Otherwise, your efforts are futile. To prevent unnecessary and unhealthy weight gain and to have a healthy nutritional lifestyle, you have to change what's happening inside your body. You need to burn fat and build lean muscle mass. Muscle is what makes you look healthy, well proportioned, and makes you feel good about your appearance. Muscle not only helps you feel good; it burns fat. The more muscle you are able to make; the more fat you will be able to burn. Don't worry, you will not look "big and bulky". Your size will go down as your muscle mass goes up, because muscle is denser than fat and takes up much less space than fat pound for pound. Remember, how we look and feel depends on our body composition which is our ratio of fat to lean mass. Ideal body composition for women is between 20 and 30% fat. Knowing that over 50% of the adult population is overweight is not surprising that most Americans are carrying at least twice as much fat as they should.

Americans are fat because they are malnourished. Malnourished in the land of plenty? Yes! Malnourished in the healthy positive partitioning agents. Protein is one of the strongest and most important positive partitioning agents. For a person to avoid fat-storage mode you should not starve or restrict your diet. Restriction further stimulates fat storage in a metabolic anticipation of a decrease in availability of nutrients. Instead, you must eat more protein, a very positive partitioning nutrient, to convert into fat burning mode. It is just that plain and simple. If you continue to eat a high carbohydrate, low-protein, low fat diet, and calorie count in an attempt to avoid excess weight, then you should expect just the opposite; you will gain weight and remain in fat storage mode. Even worse, if you lose weight, you will lose approximately 35% from lean mass and the rest from fat. When you revert back to regular eating habits, which happens most of the time because a healthy nutritional lifestyle was not established, the lost weight gets replaced primary with fat. Only about 20% lean mass gets replaced. The end effect after multiple attempts at avoiding excess weight results in muscle loss and more fat gain. Remember muscle is a major fat burner, so with each attempt and loss of muscle results in loss of fat burning capacity.

Eating enough protein prevents this. This is illustrated in a study done at Texas Christian Women's University. Two groups of middle aged obese women were put on a low-calorie diet and strength training program. Both groups were given the same number of calories. The only difference between the groups was the composition of the calories. One group ate more protein in their diet and less carbohydrates. The other group ate more carbohydrates and less protein in their diets. Both groups of women in the study lost a significant amount of weight. But, what was lost was the important difference. The low protein and high carbohydrate group lost the typical ratio of 65% fat and 35% lean mass. This ratio is typically seen in low protein and high carbohydrate diets. Fascinatingly, the weight loss by the women on the high protein and low carbohydrate diet was comprised almost exclusively of fat. The protein enriched diet, a positive partitioning agent, activated the metabolic switch to pathway A and promoted storage of lean muscle mass and inactivated the pathway B, the fat storage mode. In other words, the additional protein turned on the fat-burning metabolic pathway while promoting preservation of muscle and lean mass. The women on the high protein diet had a significant increase in their metabolic rate as compared to their low protein diet counterparts. The high protein group burned more energy and expensed more calories throughout the study than those women on low protein diets. This study perfectly illustrates the significant short comings of strict calorie cutting diets without the proper amounts of protein.

Protein is the key metabolic component in our bodies. We are designed to run on protein. There is growing evidence that ketones are also an important nutrient for our bodies and possibly preferred over carbohydrates as an energy source. Because we don't fully understand the effects of ketones in pregnancy, for now it is best to avoid this condition while you are pregnant. This is easy to do with an adequate amount of healthy carbohydrates. We will talk about what a healthy carbohydrate is in detail later on in the book.

The breakdown and absorption of food, which includes proteins, carbohydrates and fats, requires both mechanical and chemical reactions to act upon them. Mechanical action requires the activation and use of striated and smooth muscle which are composed of proteins. The biochemical reactions of metabolism are driven by protein molecules. Simply adding protein to your diet turns on the processes of fat burning and muscle building even if no other lifestyle changes are made. How much protein is enough to kick yourself into fat burning mode? I will talk about how much is enough later in the book. Sometimes, given the hectic schedule that most people keep, especially moms, it is not easy to get enough protein from food alone and a supplement maybe required.

Carbohydrates are not all bad; some can be kind. Stressing the importance of protein does not mean giving up the carbohydrates. It doesn't mean you have to cut out all the carbohydrates for a high protein diet to work. In fact, it is more important to add protein than to cut carbohydrates. When you consume a diet high in protein and low in carbohydrates you create a metabolic condition called ketosis which causes the formation of a biochemical called ketones. Ketones are substrates that are available for metabolism. When the body is not accustomed to ketones as a metabolite, they are generally eliminated rapidly from the body in the urine. Therefore, initial weight loss obtained by ketogenic diets is from loss of the body's water. Ketogenic diets also cause numerous side effects including constipation, sallow-looking skin, and a characteristic odor to the breath. Occasional and benign transient ketosis occasionally occurs during pregnancy during times of fasting and is not uncommon. It readily resolves with food intake and hydration. Ketogenic diets have raised questions about their effects on pregnancy. Animal studies with prolong exposure to ketosis during development, as would be the case in ketogenic diets, suggest abnormal development in various organ systems resulting in multiple abnormal sequel. This type of ketosis is also markedly different from that seen in ketoacidosis which can cause immediate harm to the mother and fetus. Ketosis, resulting from frank malnutrition from the unavailability of food, may be indicative of risk factors for poor fetal growth and preterm labor. These problems arising from the under lying cause and not from ketosis itself. Because the complete effects on pregnancy are unknown, animal studies suggest deleterious effects, and the lack of important carbohydrates. It is my recommendation that ketogenic diets should be avoided during pregnancy. In fact, they should probably be avoided in non-pregnant individuals except for short periods with medical management in an effort to effect a large weight loss in a short period of time. I say this because they do not provide a long term healthy nutritional lifestyle, and in time, result in an improperly balanced metabolism. Inadequate amounts of carbohydrates will prevent proper utilization of proteins and result in the inability to form muscle and stay lean.

The OB Nutritional Systems meal plan is not a ketogenic meal plan. In fact, you can eat almost unlimited amounts of good carbohydrates. Eating the good carbohydrates is important to prevent ketosis during pregnancy. Good carbohydrates are positive partitioning agents which includes most fresh fruits and vegetables. You don't have to give up all starchy carbohydrates either, like bread, potatoes and pasta. They are allowed in limited quantities. Adding protein is more important than cutting carbohydrates. I recommend a lot more protein in my meal plan, but it is done safely. Heart disease is the number one killer of women. It claims more lives in women than breast cancer and lung cancer combined. The percentage of women that die within one year of a heart attack exceeds that of men. Some people will develop atherosclerosis from a high-fat diet, so I make sure any recommendations stay well within the reasonable fat guidelines. When I recommend foods with protein I recommend ones that are low in saturated fat. Proteins low in saturated fat are good for the heart.

OB Nutritional Systems is designed to work with your metabolism. The program doesn't try to shape you up and slim you down by creating an unhealthy metabolic condition.

Instead, OB Nutritional Systems works with your metabolism, restores its balance, and promotes a healthy nutritional lifestyle. Since you are eating enough carbohydrates, you are never in ketosis and its adverse effects. I will advise you of which carbohydrates are best and instruct you to cut out all those junk carbohydrates that cause an imbalance in your metabolism. You should always feel full and satisfied and never deprived on this program.

Fiber, like protein, is another important nutrient that is needed by our bodies. Fiber is a scarce resource in our current food supply. Most people do not get enough fiber in their diet and therefore their metabolism is running less than optimal. Most people consume between 10 and 15 g of fiber a day. You should be eating at least twice that amount per day. Like protein, fiber promotes fat burning. Not surprising, protein and fiber together are one of the most powerful fat burning food combinations. Fruits and vegetables along with other good carbohydrates are an excellent source of fiber, but it is difficult for most people to get enough of them. If you're one of those people that fall in this category there are ways to supplement your fiber intake. There are several supplements available. The most common are Metamucil, Citrucel, and Fibercon.

Just say no to fructose. I am not talking about the small amounts of fructose found in fruits. Fruits have tiny amounts of pure fructose that the body can handle, along with water, fiber, vitamins, and minerals. Fruits are good for you. I am talking about the concentrated and nutritiously void fructose and high fructose corn syrup that are the primary sweeteners used in processed foods. They are also used in the frozen food industry to help prevent freezer burn. Fructose is the sneaky villain of sweeteners. Fructose does not cause as rapid of a rise in blood sugar like traditional table sugar, but it has a far more deleterious effect on metabolism. Fructose pushes your metabolism into fat storage mode and keeps it there. Fructose runs rampant throughout our food supply. If you make it a habit to read food labels you will find it listed as fructose, high fructose corn syrup, or natural fruit sweeteners. It is commonly among the first 3 to 5 ingredients listed, and if you see fructose then put it back you don't want it. You will find high fructose corn syrup just about everywhere. It is in cereals, cookies, beverages, frozen and canned goods, condiments, breakfast and nutrition bars, salad dressings, candy and desserts, and in some proclaimed health foods. Unsuspecting people probably get 15 to 20 percent of their daily calories from fructose. Kids including teenagers, probably consume more than that. I have said it once already and will likely say it again, but it's worth repeating now," just say no to fructose!"

The OB Nutritional Systems meal plan is designed to switch you from a person who stores fat to a person that burns fat. You'll put protein and fiber back into your diet and at the same time decrease starchy carbohydrates and eliminate poor carbohydrates. With each trimester you will make slight adjustments to meet nutritional requirements for that trimester of pregnancy. You should in no way feel hungry, bored, or deprived as a result of your healthy nutritional lifestyle. Some people on the program feel like they have to eat too much too often. Not eating enough food is considered cheating on this program. You only have to be concerned with tracking three nutrients: protein, fiber, and carbohydrates. I will show you how to monitor your daily consumption and provide you with charts to make it easy. When following the meal plan, keep it simple.

Most people eat the same 10 to 15 foods over and over. OB Nutritional Systems makes it easy for you to find 10 to 15 of the right foods, and of course, you can switch these around whenever you want. To simplify things more, I have assigned three ratings to food. Green foods which are the best and are all but unlimited. Yellow foods are foods which you should keep careful track of to avoid imbalances. Red foods are foods to avoid whenever possible. I will provide you with food charts to help make this simple to follow. The OB Nutritional Systems meal planner will help you keep track of what and when you are eating.

As I have said before, OB Nutritional Systems is a nutritional and fitness program which consists of five phases. The first three phases are in conjunction with the three trimesters of your pregnancy. The fourth phase focuses on the postpartum recovery and breast-feeding. The fifth phase is a maintenance phase and can be considered as a preconception phase. The meal plan and exercise method work together to produce a healthy nutritional lifestyle which is not only very effective but is also safe. There are probably several pregnant women reading this thinking you already want me to change how I eat and you want me to exercise too, who do you think you are? I am an obstetrician who has helped thousands manage their weight during pregnancy, and a person who cares about your nutritional health and how it will impact your baby and family. I know all too well that over half of pregnant women are overweight. I am sorry to say that my profession has done little to educate and take action on behalf of pregnant women in regards to nutrition. We have talked the talk, but few have walked the walk. Well, I am working on your behalf. The nutrition part of the program is by far the key to the program. In order to change your body and metabolism you have to change the way you eat. You have to eat and adapt a healthy nutritional lifestyle. You can achieve excellent results just by eating properly. But, you will get even better results and feel better if you follow both the exercise program and meal plan simultaneously.

Let's make muscle. The OB Nutritional Systems exercise plan does just that. Muscle burns fat more than any other tissue. Muscle even burns fat when your body is at rest. Our bodies are at rest approximately 70% of the time. Yes it's true you burn a lot of fat while you sleep. There's no better fat burner than muscle, and you have to exercise to make muscle. More specifically, the type of exercise needed to build muscle and lean mass is weight training. There is confusion among women that weight training will give them big, bulging muscles everywhere, while aerobics will slim them down in the right places. This is not true. Weight training does more for your body faster and better than aerobics. Aerobics does not build muscle. Aerobics turns up fat burning only during the time of exercise. When you stop aerobic exercise your fat burning ability diminishes rapidly. Weight training turns up fat burning when you exercise, but the effect continues for several days afterward. Even when you are at rest, you will still burn fat at a higher rate. The OB Nutritional Systems strength training gives your body definition not bulges. The weight training program is extremely effective and very simple.

Another great thing is that there is no huge time commitment. Which is good because I'm sure you're spending a lot of time preparing for your new baby. Hopefully, you are spending some quality time with your spouse as well since you will soon be dividing your time with another person. By the way, working out is more fun with a friend. Have your partner join you. Strength training is good for him too.

The weight training program is divided into four separate workout sessions. Each session is performed once a week and is made up five exercises. You should spend less than an hour on each session. This means your workout will take less than four hours each week. Once you have your routine down, you will likely spend no more than two hours per week completing your exercises. You can keep track of your progress with the OB Nutritional Systems workout planner. The exercises are illustrated with easy-to-follow directions. OB Nutritional Systems is designed to give you control of your body and how you look. You are establishing a healthy nutritional lifestyle that promotes building a strong healthy body, which not only feels and looks good, but gives your growing baby the best possible environment to grow healthy. You will not be depriving yourself of food, in fact you will be eating real food all day long. Best of all, you will see results and feel more energetic.

4 NUTRIENTS IN PREGNANCY

Getting the necessary nutrients, including vitamins and minerals, is important during pregnancy. I will briefly discuss a few of the more important ones. Folic acid is a B vitamin also known as folate. Studies have shown that having additional folate helps to prevent major birth defects that involve the baby's brain and spine. This class of birth defects are known as neural tube defects. It is recommended that women should take 400 micrograms of folic acid daily for a least one month prior to conception. It is also recommended that women increase their intake to 600 micrograms of folic acid daily during their pregnancy in order to reduce the risks of neural tube defects. It may be difficult to get enough folic acid from food alone. Most quality prenatal vitamins contain the proper amount of folic acid. Check the nutritional label on the vitamins to make sure there is at least 600 micrograms of folic acid. Some nutritional supplements also contain folic acid, again check the nutritional label to see how much folic acid is available. Research shows that the body absorbs the synthetic version of folic acid much better than the naturally occurring version contained in certain foods. The foods which are rich in folic acid include: lentils; dried beans and peas; dark green vegetables such as broccoli, spinach, collard or turnip greens, okra, and asparagus; and citrus fruit and juice. Food manufacturers are required by the U.S. Food and Drug Administration, in some instances, to add folic acid so that each serving contains at least 20 percent of the daily requirement. Food sources should be considered as complements to a supplement because of the limited bioavailability of their folic acid. So, the source of your folic acid, whether you get your folic acid from food, vitamins, or supplements is important to consider in making sure you get the adequate amount of 600 micrograms during the day.

Iron is another important nutrient that is difficult to get adequate amounts of during pregnancy. The body uses iron to make hemoglobin in our red blood cells. This important nutrient helps the blood cells carry oxygen to your organs and tissues. The oxygen in the blood that gets carried to the placenta gets exchanged to the fetal blood cells which carry the oxygen to your growing baby. Therefore, your body needs extra iron to make extra blood to meet all the growing demands for oxygen. The recommended daily dose of iron is twice that of a non-pregnant woman. Pregnant women should include 27 milligrams of iron in their diet every day. This is usually found in most prenatal vitamins with iron included. Again, check the nutritional label to make sure. Good sources of iron with 3.5 milligrams per serving include: clams, mollusks, mussels, and oysters. Good sources of iron with 2 milligrams per serving include: beef, sardines, turkey, apricots, and broccoli. Good sources of iron with 1 milligram per serving include: chicken, spinach, and green pepper. There are several red meats and starchy vegetables which are good sources of iron, however they are considered yellow proteins and yellow carbohydrates and should be avoided. Red meats and starchy vegetables tend to have a higher fat content and less favorable metabolic impact as compared to green proteins and green carbohydrates. Again, most dietary sources should be considered as compliments to a supplement in order to meet the daily requirements. Note: Iron absorption is improved when iron rich foods and iron supplements are eaten with vitamin C rich foods, such as citrus fruits and tomatoes.

Calcium is another important nutrient. It not only helps build teeth and bone, but calcium is essential for healthy skin and eyesight. All women, pregnant and non-pregnant, should get 1,000 milligrams of calcium daily. Those women who are 14-18 years old should get an additional 300 milligrams daily. Milk, cheese and yogurt are good sources of calcium as long as they come from the non-fat or low-fat varieties of these products. Other sources include: broccoli, leafy greens, and sardines. Of course, a calcium supplement is also available to ensure the adequate amount of calcium is consumed daily.

Vitamin D works in conjunction with calcium and it is important to get an adequate amount as well. Pregnant women and non-pregnant women need 600 international units of vitamin D daily. Good sources include low-fat or non-fat vitamin D fortified milk and salmon. Sunlight converts a chemical in the skin to vitamin D, but make sure you put on the appropriate sunscreen before going out and producing vitamin D.

Omega-3 fatty acids are an important type of fat found in many types of fish. The omega-3 fatty acids are important factors in your baby's brain development. You can easily get these nutrients by including at least 2 servings of fish in your meal plan per week. Some types of fish have higher levels of mercury. Mercury has been linked to birth defects. To avoid, or limit, mercury exposure to safe levels choose fish and shellfish such as shrimp, salmon, catfish, pollock, flounder, haddock, tilapia, sole, and ocean perch. Limit white or Albacore Tuna to 3 cans per month. Canned light tuna can be safely eaten weekly. A better alternative is canned salmon, sardines, trout, and anchovies. There are other fish that can be eaten but have higher levels of mercury and should be limited to no more than six 6-ounce servings per month. These include: halibut, carp, snapper, cod, freshwater perch, bass, lobster, and mahi mahi. Because of unsafe levels of mercury you should avoid: shark, swordfish, tilefish, king mackerel, orange roughy, marlin, bigeye tuna and Ahi tuna. As with most other vitamins, there are supplemental forms available for the omega-3 fatty acids.

There are several other vitamins and minerals which are important and can easily be obtained by eating a well-rounded diet. Taking a prenatal vitamin daily will ensure that you are getting those extra vitamins and minerals. Oils and fats are also important nutrients in limited amounts and are easily obtained from the lean proteins and healthy plant sources you will find in your meal plan.

The last nutritional issue I want to discuss is in regards to caloric needs and healthy weight gain during pregnancy. What comprises the additional calories required during pregnancy will likely surprise you; it did me. You have likely heard someone say that they are eating for two. That is not quite true. Yes there are two people, but one of them is much smaller. In fact, there is no additional calorie requirement for the first trimester. The second trimester requires an additional 150 calories daily and the third trimester another 150 calories for a total of 300 additional calories daily. This is the equivalent to 1.5 apples daily for the second trimester and 3 apples daily in the third trimester. Alternately, how about 5 graham crackers or 16 animal crackers the second trimester and 10 graham crackers or 32 animal crackers the third trimester. It does not seem that much when you think of it in terms of food items. Why then do so many pregnant women justify eating that milk shake, dessert, and many other things by saying they are eating for two? The fact is most people just don't know better.

The current recommended caloric requirement for pregnancy is based on a woman's starting BMI, or body mass index. The baseline, or neutral, calorie requirement for her BMI is required for the first trimester; baseline plus 150 calories for the second trimester; baseline plus 300 calories for the third trimester. The baseline calorie requirement, theoretically, is the amount of calories required for a given BMI so that there is a neutral change in weight. In other words, there is no increase or decrease in weight. Therefore, the only time I will be concerned about calories is while you are pregnant. I am not worried about you getting too many calories, I just want to make sure that you get enough calories for your stage of pregnancy. When you are no longer pregnant, you do not have to track calories. If you remember, the quality of the foods is much more important than the quantity. In fact, you can consume much more calories than are required as long as they are from the right food groups, the Green groups. When you stay within the Green groups you will not gain any unnecessary or unhealthy weight while you are pregnant.

5 WEIGHT GAIN AND PREGNANCY

Now that we have mentioned weight, let's talk about weight gain. The American College of Obstetricians and Gynecologists follows the Institute of Medicine recommendations with regard to weight gain during pregnancy. These recommendations are as follows: underweight women or BMI<18.5 should gain between 28-40 pounds, normal weight women or BMI 18.5-24.9 should gain between 25-30 pounds, overweight women or BMI 25-29.9 should gain between 15-25 pounds, and obese women or BMI 30 and greater should gain between 11-20 pounds. I have read the report and recommendations by the Institute of Medicine, and I have read the committee opinion published by the American College of Obstetricians and Gynecologists with regards to weight gain during pregnancy. To better understand these recommendations, you have to first understand the committee's process. They have to take in consideration multiple factors and opinions, and at best, it is a compromise of many various opinions. I do not fully agree with the recommendations because of its predetermined amount of weight gain based on a total weight of a single system. It does not consider the mother and pregnancy as separate systems. I consider this as arbitrary and do not take in account a net difference between two systems.

The American College of Obstetricians and Gynecologists clearly state in their committee opinion that the Institute of Medicine recommendations have also met with controversial reactions from some physicians who also feel the weight gain targets are too high. The American College of Obstetricians and Gynecologists, in their summary, does recognize that individualized care and clinical judgment are necessary in managing a woman who is gaining less weight than recommended but has an appropriately growing fetus. I strongly agree with this point. Let me tell you why. When you consider the weight gain during pregnancy you have to consider what makes up that weight gain. The weight gain or loss is the net total from two systems. The mother makes up one system, and the developing baby makes up the second system. To keep things simple, the developing baby is considered to be all associated pregnancy changes including the fetus, placenta, increased blood and fluid volume, and other pregnancy associated changes. The mother's system, when subjected to a healthy nutritional lifestyle, will begin building lean muscle mass and

24

burning off fat regardless of the amount of calories taken in. The body is no longer storing fat, it is moving it out and burning it off. It is not doing this because of dieting or a lack of nutrition. It is doing this because it is being feed the right nutrition and her metabolism is running very efficiently. Therefore, the mother's system can actually lose several pounds of fat over a nine month period, while the baby's system gains the appropriate amount of weight.

For example, a pregnant woman is 5 feet 6 inches tall and weighs 200 pounds at the start of her pregnancy. This gives her a BMI of 32, which is considered obese. Let's assume the mother's system losses 2 pounds per week with a healthy nutritional lifestyle for a total of 80 pounds during the 40 weeks of gestation. Let's assume the pregnancy system gains an appropriate 30 pounds. This would give a net loss of 50 pounds with a normal and appropriately growing fetus. This is what should be considered normal! If you blindly followed the Institute of Medicine recommendations for this same woman and encouraged her to gain 10-20 pounds during her pregnancy then she would be 220 pounds at the end of 40 weeks. Instead of being a healthier 150 pounds with a normal BMI of 24 post-delivery, she would be 220 with a BMI now over 35. Let me point out here the physician's Hippocratic Oath! First, do no harm! No wonder the medical profession is failing two thirds of the pregnant women, we are giving them the wrong information.

I selected 100 patients in my practice with similar BMI's, races and social economic backgrounds. The BMI's ranged between 25 and 30. I choose this range to avoid including any natural genetic fat burners. In group 1, I had 50 of the patients keep a food diary for me to review during their pregnancy and gave them general nutritional and exercise recommendations without specific instructions. In group 2, I made nutritional recommendations to 50 of the patients that included eating a healthy nutritional diet with increased portions of proteins, keeping to healthy Green carbohydrates, and added an exercise regimen during their pregnancy. I also discussed nutritional and exercise issues in depth at each visit and went over their food diary each visit as well. I had about half of the group 1 patients keep up their food diaries enough to assess completely their nutritional picture. The other half either did not complete the dairies enough or frequently "forgot them" and therefore were excluded. One individual in Group 1 developed gestational diabetes and was excluded for treatment. The entire Group 1, as I expected, had a typical western diet high in carbohydrates and low in protein. Group 2, had a similar compliance rate as Group 1. Twenty women in Group 2 actually kept their diaries consistently and correctly. Of these twenty, 10 women were compliant enough with instructions for the diet recommendations and exercise regimen to be included. In Group 1, the range of weight gain was 20 to 60 pounds with an average of a 38 pound weight gain. The average fetal weight for Group 1 was 7 pounds and 14 ounces. In Group 2, the range of weight gain was -15 pounds to +10 pounds with an average of a 5 pound weight gain. The average fetal weight for Group 2 was 7 pounds and 2 ounces. Group 1 had four cesarean sections. One for non-reassuring fetal heart tones and three for failure to progress. Group 1 had three vacuum assists to affect delivery. Group 1 also had a few mild vaginal and perineal lacerations, but five required repair. One with a partial third degree tear. Group 1 had on average longer labors and longer duration of pushing to accomplish delivery. One member of Group 1 was removed because of gestational diabetes. The average hospital stay for Group 1 was 1.5 days.

Group 2 had uncomplicated labors and spontaneous deliveries without vacuum or forceps assistance. There was only a few mild vaginal and perineal lacerations. With one primary laceration requiring repair. No cesarean sections, episiotomies, extended tears, extended labors or extended pushing or gestation diabetes in Group 2. All members of group 2 were discharged within 24 hours. This small observational study I performed suggests the importance of nutrition and exercise for both mom and baby, and the importance of maintaining a healthy nutritional lifestyle during pregnancy. A healthy nutritional lifestyle not only improves outcomes and decreases hospitalization time but provides overall better outcomes. The women feel better, have more energy, have an overall positive attitude, and prove to have more rewarding experiences.

This observational study warrants the need for a large randomized study to help shed light on the issue of obesity in pregnant women and to allow appropriate recommendations by the Institute of Medicine and give the American College of Obstetricians and Gynecologists the needed clinical evidence to guide them on making clear and direct recommendations for providers to follow.

The American College of Obstetricians and Gynecologists in their committee opinion does state that providers who care for pregnant women should determine their BMI as part of their initial prenatal visit. It also states that she should be counseled about nutrition and exercise and what constitutes healthy and appropriate weight gain. Especially important is a discussion of limiting and avoiding excess weight gain to achieve best pregnancy outcomes. I have talked to numerous women about whether or not they had any significant discussion with their obstetrician or provider with regards to nutrition and exercise during pregnancy. None of the women I talked to had any significant discussion with regard to nutrition. Those that directly asked about exercise where given vague instructions and mainly told to just keep doing what they were already doing. Giving no information is just as wrong as giving bad information in my opinion. I understand why most obstetricians don't discuss nutrition and exercise, but it is not excusable. Most of the time, they not only lack the knowledge but also lack the time. Most practices are under time and billing pressures and most reimbursements don't pay for the necessary additional time for nutritional and exercise counseling. Surprisingly, nutrition and physical exercise are not formally taught in medical school and residency, so nutritional and exercise experience among providers will vary extensively. Unfortunately, their recommendations will be what they learned to be normal, which is what they grew up with, and will most likely mirror the current western diet of high carbohydrates and low protein. I am afraid until we make a significant impact on overweight and obesity issues during pregnancy we will not make any progress in reducing their associated complications.

6 WHY OB NUTRITIONAL SYSTEMS WORKS

The key to understanding how and why OB Nutritional Systems works is to understand the biochemistry of metabolism and energy production. Metabolism and energy production are the results of several different types of biochemical reactions. Some reactions are spontaneous, that is whenever the needed substrates are present they react together. This reaction maybe slow or fast. Some reactions require energy to initiate the reaction process. Still other reactions require enzymes, or coenzymes, to enable a reaction to occur. Some reactions go forward or reverse depending on the concentrations of the substrates. Some reactions are not reversible. Combining all these reactions in various ways allows a cell or organism to control or limit the metabolic process depending on the condition presented to the cell. The metabolic process can be either catabolic or anabolic. Catabolic processes breakdown molecules for energy. Anabolic processes build up cells or store molecules. I will talk about breaking down molecules for energy first.

I will start with a carbohydrate. The carbohydrate enters the cell as glucose and then starts down the metabolic pathway. The first phase in the process of glycolysis then occurs. Glycolysis refers to the process of metabolizing glucose and it occurs in two phases. A few key things happen here. The glucose is immediately phosphorylated. This reaction is not easy to reverse and it prevents the glucose from exiting the cell. In phase one, a reaction occurs with a regulatory enzyme called phosphofructokinase. This enzyme is activated by AMP and inhibited by ATP. ATP is the body's key energy molecule. As the ATP molecule is used it is converted to AMP. As energy needs increase the enzyme is activated, and as energy needs decrease the enzyme is deactivated. This is the major regulatory step in glycolysis. The next phase results in a final and irreversible step which subsequently results in conversion of glucose into 2 molecules of pyruvate. The pyruvate gets converted to acetyl-CoA and enters the Krebs cycle, and through a series of reactions is further metabolized. This complete process from glucose to pyruvate and complete metabolism results in the production of 36 molecules of ATP.

When proteins are metabolized for energy they first go through a process to remove the amino group. This process is called transamination, which is the transfer of an amino group from one molecule to another. The resulting amino acids enter the metabolic pathway at several various points depending on the amino acid. Some enter as pyruvate and acetyl-CoA. Others enter as one of four intermediaries along the Kreb's cycle.

When fat is metabolized, it under goes a series of reactions known as β-oxidation. This breaks down the fatty acid molecule. The initiation of fatty acid oxidation requires activation of the relatively unreactive fatty acid molecule. The unreactive nature explains why fat is so difficult to get rid of. The activated form is similar to acetyl-CoA and the fatty acid byproducts of the β-oxidation enter the metabolic pathway as acetyl-CoA.

Now, I will talk about building up cells and storing energy. The body is constantly in a state of change. The body is growing, repairing, protecting, storing, regulating, and moving. It is also communicating and transporting between cells. This is the work of proteins. The cells use a process called protein synthesis to build and interact the various proteins in order to accomplish these tasks. This is also the process used to build lean muscle mass, which you should remember is a major fat burner. When we strength train we stimulate this process. Muscle is also a place to store energy. The body rapidly and quickly utilizes protein for energy when in a fasting state. That is why it is important to eat all throughout the day and eat frequently. You should start getting an appreciation of the demand for protein, if you haven't already.

The production of fatty acids is necessary to form the membrane lipids of cells, but the main reason for the production of fatty acids is to convert excess dietary carbohydrates to fats for storage. The key molecule for this process is acetyl-CoA. The key enzymes are acetyl-CoA carboxylase and a complex referred to as fatty acid synthase. When an increase in carbohydrate, or glucose, levels occur, a corresponding increase in insulin occurs. The release of insulin triggers a series of steps that results in the activation of acetyl-CoA carboxylase, the key enzyme in fat storage.

This is a simplified description of what happens; it occurs in all the cells all throughout the body. In addition, cells of various organs and tissues may be more or less metabolically active depending on the biologic activity going on. Certain cells, tissues, and organs are also more specialized for certain processes as well. But this should give you a rough picture of what is going on metabolically.

First, let us look at how this system was meant to work. Remember, for an organism to survive it must be able to adapt to its environment. Whether you are a creationist or evolutionist we had to start somewhere and had to eat something. So, we can all agree it started a very long time ago and we had to eat what was available at that time. It is safe to say there were no grocery stores, restaurants, or processed foods available in the early times. We had to eat whatever we caught or found. The major food source in our diets at that time would have been lean protein from the animals or fish that we caught. This high protein diet was complimented by fresh high fiber carbohydrates. The carbohydrates would have included raw vegetables, edible grasses, raw nuts, and an occasional piece of fruit when in season. It is likely they ate roughly the same quantity, but definitely not the same quality of carbohydrates we do today. Our ancestors had a much higher quality of carbohydrate. This diet was mainstay for thousands of years, until we became more of an agricultural society starting about 10,000 years ago. Let's see how this diet interacts with our metabolism.

Let's look at protein. The protein can be readily and freely used for anabolic functions and catabolic functions. The proteins can enter the metabolic pathway at several points and are for the most part concentration driven reactions. The carbohydrates must enter at the beginning of the metabolic pathway and must follow along the pathway in a sequential order. Since all the carbohydrates available to our ancestors had a low metabolic impact. They were all considered Green carbohydrates, or positive partitioning agents. They did not cause an excessive or prolonged increase in insulin levels. Why is this important? Remember, the release of insulin triggers a series of steps that turns on and activates the key enzyme responsible for fat storage. If you have an excessive increase in insulin you increase the signal to store fat. Insulin also stimulates glucose into the cells. With high levels of insulin, the glucose is being crowed into the cell which is being stimulated to store the excess carbohydrates into fat. A normal insulin response moves glucose into the cells with minimal stimulation of fat promoting enzymes, so it can be metabolized and used as energy instead of being stored. This reinforces and supplements the energy being produced from protein. Therefore, it allows more protein for anabolic needs. It is also important to note, since most of what we ate came in the form of protein, the majority of our nutrients presented themselves for metabolism into the Krebs cycle and not in glycolysis. This results in less substrate available for fatty acid production. Remember, a large number of biochemical reactions are concentration driven or regulated.

With the development of agriculture approximately 10,000 years ago, came a slight shift in the composition of our diets. Breads, grains, and starches become more prevalent in the diets because of their convenience. They were easier to grow and store than other sources and they were also tasty and filling. These new food sources displaced some of the previous proteins and high fiber grasses and vegetables. A comparison of societies from these two eras shows how diets impact our health. People from the agricultural era were heavier than their predecessors and began showing evidence of dental cavities, heart disease and diabetes. What happened along the metabolic pathway? Proportionately more nutrients introduced through glycolysis than directly into the Kreb cycle. In other words, More carbohydrates and less protein. The new carbohydrates had a greater metabolic impact and caused increased insulin responses. This results in more substrates available for fat storage and increased insulin activity which increases acetyl-CoA carboxylase activity. Remember this enzyme is the key enzyme for fat storage. This explains why people from the agricultural area as a whole were a fatter society as compared to their ancestors.

Now, let's look at what has happened over the past few decades since 1960. The western diet has become a predominately carbohydrate and highly processed diet severely depleted of protein. Nutrition has given way to extended shelf life, easy shipping and convenience. Carbohydrates are crammed down an overloaded glycolysis. The Kreb cycle is void of amino acids. The acetyl-CoA carboxylase, aka the fat enzyme, is now in overdrive. This is in a non-pregnant person. Imagine what happens when this same person is now pregnant.

During pregnancy there is a significant increase in various hormones including cortisol, estrogen, and progesterone. There is also a change in metabolism that serves to shunt nutrients to the fetus. This is accomplished by a gradual increase in insulin resistance as pregnancy progresses, and results in a hyperinsulinemic-euglycemic state. Under the influence of the previously mentioned hormones, this metabolic state favors lipogenesis and fat storage. This metabolic design occurred in a setting of high protein and high quality high fiber carbohydrates. Under these conditions, there is plenty of protein to provide a supply of amino acids for fetal development and maternal needs. The carbohydrates being consumed have a low metabolic impact and have little impact on insulin or fat storage. The insulin resistance produced by the pregnancy hormones was actually needed to appropriately shunt nutrients to the developing fetus after ingestion of meals. The insulin resistance also insures gluconeogenesis, by the liver, between ingestion of meals. This allows a consistent flow of nutrients to the developing baby. The metabolism fits the nutrition in these conditions.

Now, with today's pregnancy and today's diet, there is a large mismatch. There is a disproportionate amount of poor quality carbohydrates being presented to the pregnant metabolic system. Like the non-pregnant state, the carbohydrates are overloaded into glycolysis but now there is a hormone induced insulin resistance. The two of these coupled together further the lipogenic state and fat storage. At the same time the pathway for protein is underutilized. Continuing the modern western diet while pregnant is a recipe for disaster.

OB Nutritional Systems is no big secret, nor is it some magical pill. The program brings to your pregnancy the nutritional elements that it was designed for. That is why it works. It works with your metabolism instead of sabotaging it. You can think of OB Nutritional Systems as your metabolic matchmaker.

7 WEIGHT AND PREGNANCY COMPLICATIONS

Overweight and obese women are at an increased risk of several pregnancy problems and complications. The most common pregnancy problems include gestational diabetes, high blood pressure and cesarean delivery. More serious pregnancy problems include preeclampsia and preterm labor. Gestational diabetes is a type of diabetes that develops, or is diagnosed in women for the first time during their pregnancy. You usually get screened between 24 and 28 weeks gestation. You may get screened sooner if you have risk factors for diabetes. Risk factors for diabetes include: overweight and obese individuals, previous gestational diabetes, history of having a very large baby, having a previous unexplained stillbirth, and a first degree relative with diabetes. Gestational diabetes, like diabetes mellitus, is a condition that causes higher than normal levels of glucose in the blood. Having too high of a blood glucose level can cause health problems to occur. Gestational diabetes occurs when a woman's body responds abnormally to the hormone insulin. Insulin moves glucose from the blood to the various cells and tissues to be used. During pregnancy, the woman's cells normally become slightly resistant to the effects of insulin, resulting in a slightly higher level of glucose in the blood. This can provide more nutrients to the growing baby. In response, the mother's body makes slightly more insulin to keep the blood glucose level normal. However, in some women the increased level in insulin cannot keep the blood glucose within a normal range resulting in gestational diabetes. Women who develop gestational diabetes during pregnancy have almost a 50% chance of developing type II diabetes later on in life. These women should also be screened for diabetes after the postpartum period and again every few years. Gestational diabetes complicates pregnancies by causing an increase in the risk of having a very large baby, a fetal demise, possible pelvic floor injuries, a cesarean section, hypertension, and preeclampsia.

Babies born to mothers with gestational diabetes are at risk for low glucose levels, jaundice, and may even have problems with breathing. Gestational diabetes also increases the risk of delivery complications including shoulder dystocia which can result in birth injury to the baby. Babies born to mothers with gestational diabetes are at higher risk for developing diabetes and should be monitored for diabetes risks. It is important to note, these same risks of excessive growth, birth defects, birth injuries and childhood obesity also occur in babies of overweight and obese mothers without gestational diabetes.

Blood pressure in our bodies results from a complex interaction of inputs involving the heart, nervous system, and blood vessels. Particularly, the smaller arteries. In people with high blood pressure, or hypertension, there is an abnormal amount of tightening in the arteries which causes an increase in blood pressure. One of the most common causes of high blood pressure is being overweight or obese. Losing weight and exercise can help reduce or eliminate high blood pressure. Some people have to take medications to keep their blood pressure at safe levels. Mothers with high blood pressure during their pregnancy may have a decreased amount of blood flow to the placenta, which can result in poor growth of their baby. When high blood pressure, without any other findings, first occurs during pregnancy it is called gestational hypertension, or pregnancy induced hypertension. This usually warrants closer monitoring and resolves soon after delivery.

When pregnancy induced hypertension occurs with other findings including: protein in the urine and swelling of the face and hands it is called preeclampsia. Preeclampsia is a serious condition which affects multiple organ systems, particularly the kidneys. Nonspecific signs of preeclampsia include visual disturbances and headaches. Rapid weight gain can also proceed, or coincide, with the development of preeclampsia. The exact cause of preeclampsia is unknown. But there are multiple risk factors which include: first pregnancy, history of preeclampsia, advanced maternal age, chronic hypertension, obesity, diabetes, renal disease, and certain autoimmune disorders. If a woman develops preeclampsia, she is usually hospitalized and monitored along with the baby. The only cure for preeclampsia is delivery. The decision to deliver will be made by your provider and depends on several factors including: the risks to you and the baby, how early you are, and the severity or progression of the preeclampsia. Regardless, the end goal will be to deliver the baby in order to prevent a condition called eclampsia.

Eclampsia results from the development of seizures in women with preeclampsia. Delivery may occur by vaginal delivery or by cesarean section depending on the health and condition of the mother and baby. During the labor and delivery process you may be given medications to help prevent seizures and or to decrease your blood pressure.

The increase in preterm birth in overweight and obese women is typically a result of problems and complications related to gestational diabetes, hypertension, and preeclampsia. Cesarean section delivery is also increased among overweight and obese women. This is related to the increased risk of other pregnancy related problems including hypertension, preeclampsia, and gestational diabetes. Women with gestational diabetes as well as overweight and obese women without diabetes are at risk for having excessively large babies. These large babies result in difficulties with vaginal delivery and progression of labor, which results in an increased risk for having a cesarean section. Overweight and obese women are also at increased risk for numerous post-delivery complications including infection, deep vein thrombosis, and extended hospitalizations. The best way to reduce all these problems, risks, and complications is to effect a change that will help reduce excessive weight among our expecting mothers. We have identified the problem, and we can provide these women with a solution. The solution is to adopt a healthy nutritional lifestyle.

There is a particular group of pregnant women, which reducing risks is especially important during their pregnancies. I feel it would be appropriate at this time to talk about them briefly. There are a significant number of women who plan to attempt a vaginal birth after having a cesarean section known as a VBAC. There are a significant number of women who participate in home births. I understand the multiple reasons and motivations these women have to pursue these options. The women who plan to VBAC or have home births need to reduce their risk factors as much as possible to increase their chances of a successful outcome. Following OB Nutritional Systems and maintaining a healthy nutritional lifestyle will prevent unnecessary weight gain. Overweight and obese patients may actually result in a healthy net loss in weight and therefore reduce the risks associated with an overweight pregnancy. The reduction of these associated risks may make a difference when it comes to having a successful outcome.

8 FETAL MONITORING AND WELLBEING

I recommend this program for you, so you can obtain and maintain a healthy nutritional lifestyle, which should have a positive influence on you, your pregnancy and your family. Just as important as healthy nutrition, you should have early and regular prenatal care. A discussion with your prenatal care provider, will help you determine whether or not you have any specific risk factors or weight issues that need to be addressed. We all benefit from healthy nutrition, but discuss this program with your prenatal care provider to determine if you have any special medical problems or concerns that may prevent or limit your use of this program. The two of you can decide whether this program or a program your provider outlines is best for you. Your provider will like knowing that you are taking an active part in your prenatal nutrition. The two of you together can determine the best way to monitor your pregnancy's growth and progress. I like a healthy discussion about nutrition with my patients, which includes how I plan to monitor their progress.

The best way to keep your baby healthy is to keep yourself healthy. I have mentioned this several times by now, and this is done by eating healthy. In the process of eating healthy, your body will burn off unnecessary weight from fat and avoid unnecessary weight gain. Shedding excess weight helps reduce associated risk factors during your pregnancy. This weight loss can be significant when you are overweight or obese. Providers and expecting moms are not accustomed to this weight loss, even though the baby is growing and developing normally. Since they cannot directly see the developing baby, the concern for expecting moms and providers is whether the baby is growing properly and doing well. This reassurance is easily obtained by monitoring the growing baby. There are six common methods to monitor and determine fetal wellbeing. Three of these methods do not require special equipment and include: fetal kick counts, Leopold's maneuver, and fundal height measurements. The other three methods, still easy to perform, but require special equipment and training include: fetal non-stress test, ultrasound measurements of the fetus, and ultrasound measurements of the amniotic fluid index.

Fetal kick counts are performed by the expecting mom. You perform these counts by monitoring the fetal movements, which may include: kicks, rolls, swishes, stretches, and jabs. You should count at least ten movements within an hour. If not, monitor for an additional hour. If you do not get ten movements in that second hour, you should contact your provider immediately for further evaluation. Also, if you notice a significant decrease in the regular fetal movement counts contact your provider. I recommend my patients, both high and low risk, to start doing kick counts three times per day starting with the 28th week of gestation. Regular and consistent fetal movement suggests fetal wellbeing and is reassuring to both the mom and provider.

Fundal height measurement, and the Leopold's maneuver is performed by your provider. The Leopold's maneuver is used to determine the position of the fetus and is a crude method to estimate fetal weight. The maneuver involves four distinct actions performed on the maternal abdomen around the gravid uterus. This method is mainly used to quickly determine fetal position and a rough estimate of size when ultrasound is unavailable. The fundal height measurement involves measuring the distance in centimeters from the top of the pubic bone to the top of the uterus with a simple measuring tape. After 20 weeks gestation, the distance in centimeters roughly coincides with the gestational week of the pregnancy. When the measurement and gestational age coincide, it suggests normal growth and fetal wellbeing. A larger or smaller measurement may suggest the baby is growing abnormally small or abnormally large. These findings warrant further evaluation by ultrasound. Fundal height measurement can be difficult to use on overweight or obsess women. This measurement technique is simple to perform, but can also be less accurate.

The fetal non-stress test involves using a special piece of equipment called a cardiotocograph. It records and graphs the fetal heart rate and monitors for uterine contractions. The test is used to assess the presence of two episodes of fetal heart rate accelerations within a twenty minute time period. If this occurs, the test is considered to be reactive, and provides reassurance of fetal wellbeing. In the absence of accelerations, the test is considered non-reactive and further evaluation is performed. The test is performed and read under the direction of your provider. The test is easy to perform and is non-invasive. I use this test routinely, throughout the pregnancies on both my high and low risk patients.

Ultrasound testing also requires a special piece of equipment and training. The ultrasound machine can give you and your provider a lot of valuable information. The fetal anatomy can be evaluated for birth defects by visualization obtained by using the ultrasound equipment. The location and condition of the placenta can be determined. The position of the fetus can also be determined. The gestational age can be confirmed and the growth of the fetus can be assessed by ultrasound examination. This is done by taking several fetal measurements which include the following: bi-parietal diameter, head circumference, abdominal circumference, and femur length. These measurements are compared and combined to obtain an estimated fetal weight and age. It also compares the head and abdomen for symmetrical growth. Abnormal values or abnormal comparisons may indicate further evaluation to determine the specific cause. The amniotic fluid index can also be calculated. This is done by measuring a vertical pocket of amniotic fluid in each of the four quadrants of the gravid uterus. A decrease in the amniotic fluid index usually precedes, but not always, growth related problems. A low amniotic fluid index may indicate further evaluation or monitoring. All of this information can be obtained easily and readily by performing an ultrasound examination.

Evaluation of fetal growth and wellbeing is important to document in all pregnancies. It is especially important to have that reassurance when a healthy net loss in weight is occurring. A healthy net loss in weight occurs when the maternal compartment of the pregnancy loses more weight than the fetal compartment gains; this weight loss being the result of your body burning off excess fat as a result of maintaining a healthy nutritional lifestyle. I recommend and perform ultrasounds every 2 to 4 weeks to evaluate and determine an estimated fetal weight. By obtaining serial examinations for estimated fetal weight, your provider can establish a growth curve for the developing fetus. This information will provide reassurance of normal fetal growth, or will alert your provider of a developing problem. In conjunction with determining an estimated fetal weight, I assess the amniotic fluid index. Normal findings of the estimated fetal weight, growth curve, and amniotic fluid index provide the necessary reassurance of fetal growth that you and your provider need and want.

9 OB NUTRITIONAL SYSTEMS MEAL PLAN

The Secrets for Success

The key to being successful is to have a good plan or strategy. This is true for everything we do, or are involved in. People don't plan to fail; they fail to plan. So, let's talk about some important strategies that we use to succeed in obtaining a healthy nutritional lifestyle during your pregnancy. Strategies that we will incorporate into the meal plan to help you gain healthy pregnancy weight, prevent unnecessary weight gain, and loose some of the extra fat that you might be carrying now. The strategy used by OB Nutritional Systems has multiple components which we will prioritize and discuss.

The number one priority is food. Food is the raw materials that your body metabolizes and then uses. If you provide the body with good quality nutritious food, then your body will build lean muscle and burn fat. If you give your body poor quality less nutritious food, then the body works against itself and begins to largely store fat. To achieve a stronger, leaner, and healthier body, you must give it the right foods. If you do nothing else but change the foods you eat, you will get results. Results that not only make you look and feel better, but results that are healthy. Good food is key to good health which is also key to a healthy pregnancy. Also, don't forget, a healthy nutritional lifestyle is one of the most important factors in avoiding pregnancy related complications now, and heart disease, high blood pressure and diabetes in the future. Make food your number one priority for the health of it.

The second priority is to eat enough food and to eat it often. Do you ever wonder where three scheduled meals a day came from? No other animal except man has breakfast, lunch and dinner. Instead animals eat all day long whenever they are hungry. We too should be eating all throughout the day and whenever we are hungry. You should divide your daily intake into six or more mini meals. This provides your body with a steady stream of nutritious food which keeps it burning fat and building muscle. Your metabolism works much better when it is fed a steady stream of quality nutrients. When you skip meals and cut calories it disrupts your metabolism, and you disrupt fat burning. The less frequently you eat, the more likely your body is to store fat. At first you may think eating six meals a day is hard to do, and that you don't have time. Not true. Having cared for thousands of pregnant women, I know for a fact they like food. They also typically eat all throughout the day. This makes pregnant women a natural for this program. They just need to change what they are eating. Most people that eat only three meals a day usually find themselves picking up snacks and things and eating them throughout the day anyway. The problem is, the food being snacked on is usually poor quality junk food. With no effort at all you can easily make a habit out of eating six nutritious meals scattered throughout the day and eating more whenever you are hungry. The key is to make those mini-meals work for you and not against you. This is where OB Nutritional Systems Meal Plan will help you. It will help you learn how to eat six meals of the right foods.

Another key strategy for success is keeping good successful people working for you. In this case, I am referring to protein and fiber. They are the good, successful and hardworking friends you will have working for you. Protein and fiber will transition your current body into a strong lean body and keep it there if you let them. Building muscle at the expense of fat requires adequate amounts of both protein and fiber. Make sure your strategy includes eating adequate amounts of high quality lean proteins and fiber-rich foods. Protein provides the necessary nutrients you need to operate an efficient metabolism and to build, operate, and repair other parts of your body, including your pregnancy. Fiber not only stimulates fat burning it counteracts the damaging effects of some of the less nutritious carbohydrates and helps in the elimination of toxins. Protein and fiber are the good guys, so keep them close and in good quality and quantity.

A good book always needs a villain. In our book, the villain's name is Fructose, aka High Fructose Corn syrup. Obviously our next strategic priority is to stay away from the villain Fructose. Don't be fooled by his popularity and celebrity status among our food supply. He might look sweet and taste sweet but fructose is anything but sweet when it comes to destroying your metabolism, storing fat, and subsequently giving your pregnancy unwanted and unhealthy weight gain. Just because fructose is a popular ingredient among food manufactures and commonly found in all sorts of food at our markets, does not mean you have to buy it. Not only do you not have to buy, you don't have to eat, serve, or cook with products that contain a high amount of fructose. Fructose lurks in all sorts of food, especially the prepared and processed snacks that are marketed to children. It is no wonder that obesity has become a problem in childhood as well as adults. As a result, obesity in children has become one of the fastest growing pediatric problems in America. In my opinion, all the presweetened processed junk food directed towards children are the real child predators. Make a habit of reading the nutritional labels on foods and identifying those with fructose before you put them in your basket. You will quickly start to recognize all the places the villain likes to hang out. If the product contains fructose then put it back on the shelf and leave it. You should also keep your children or future child fructose-free, except for the tiny amounts of natural fructose found in fresh fruits. The body can handle those small amounts, and also gets the benefit of all the nutritious aspects of the fruit. Keeping your children free of fructose will be a major step in helping them to avoid childhood obesity and serious metabolic problems as they grow up. Fructose, like other villains, has an accomplice. His accomplice is the slightly less dastardly Sucrose, avoid him as much as possible too.

The last to prioritize is a simple one. Yes, keep it simple. Having worked with thousands of patients and countless others over the years the one thing that has always been true is to keep it simple. Patients are far more compliant when things are kept simple. Especially when you are asking them to make new healthier lifestyle changes. They are having a hard enough time breaking and unlearning old habits. Don't complicate things by asking them to do new complex things too. The good news, people naturally simplify their diets. Most people eat the same twelve to fifteen foods over and over again, day after day. The problem is that they eat the wrong twelve to fifteen foods. The strategy or goal of OB Nutritional Systems is to make it easy for you to switch the bad choices for good choices. With the help from the mini-meal planner you will create a simple list of ten to fifteen favorite foods from a list of high quality proteins and carbohydrates. From these favorites, you will then design your daily diet. Everyone likes variety, but simplicity rules. When confronted with too many choices, people tend to get confused and frustrated and then stop being compliant or just quit all together. I know pregnant women frequently have changes in food preferences, so I have designed the favorites section to be updated at each trimester. But, you can make more frequent substitutions if preferences occurring in pregnancy override. All I ask is to keep it simple, and you will succeed.

What You Need to Know

The OB Nutritional System Meal Plan is divided into five phases. These phases include the three trimesters of pregnancy, a postpartum recovery period, and a maintenance phase. The meal plan will allow for a wide variety of tastes and styles. You can design your meals around the foods you like. The great thing about the meal plans is that you can design them to fit your lifestyle. The plan works if you want to prepare all your meals at home, but will work equally well if you are on the run. Being a busy obstetrician and having seven kids, I know all about on the run. I follow the same meal plan as in the maintenance phase, and more than half my meals are in the truck, hospital, ball field, school functions, etc. I think you get the picture. If I can stay on track I know you can. The key is to have a plan. Through the OB Nutritional Systems Meal Planner, I will guide you through the process much like I do with by patients in the office. The planner contains all the information you will need to customize the meal plan to make it work for you. At the beginning of that section you will find a detailed step by step description of the process. This includes how to complete each part and what order to complete the forms so that you won't have any difficulty. The OB Nutritional Systems Food Charts contain the lists of proteins and carbohydrates that you can choose from to create the daily meal selections you want. The proteins and carbohydrates are listed separately and each subdivided into three different categories. The categories are Green, Yellow, and Red and the color corresponds to the quality of the proteins and carbohydrates.

Green Means Good! These are the good guys. They will help you gain healthy pregnancy weight and prevent unnecessary weight gain. The Green proteins and carbohydrates are the healthiest and the most efficient fat burners. These foods should be sought after in abundance. The Green proteins include the leanest cuts of meat and fish. They also include non-fat and low-fat dairy products. Among the good guys you will find an occasional super hero.

Likewise, among the Green proteins you will have the super hero equivalents called Super Green proteins. Super Green proteins are the lowest in fat content. They include most white meat poultry, game meat, fish, and low-fat, non-fat cottage cheese. If you already have a high amount of body fat or have a strong history of heart disease in your family you may want to make most of your protein selections from the Super Green group. Also, if you are going for the super cut look, stay with the Super Greens. The Super Green proteins are indicated by an asterisk in the charts. Those moms to be that have moderate to average body fat, are already lean, or are wanting to maintain or improve their current level of fitness, can eat freely from any of the Green proteins.

Green carbohydrates include a large assortment of fruits, vegetables, and two high fiber cereals. The Green carbohydrates are your primary source of fiber and also prevent ketosis from occurring. You can and should eat as many Green carbohydrates as you want! Green carbohydrates are your all you can eat buffet!

Remember at the beginning of this section we talked about strategy? The first two priorities were food and eat enough often. Seriously, the only way you will not be successful with this program is if you do not eat your daily requirements of Green and Super Green foods. These foods allow your metabolism to run smooth and efficient. I don't like to be hungry, and I know my patients don't like to be hungry. You shouldn't be hungry either, and you won't if you meet your daily requirements. The only reason I have you track your calories is to make sure you get enough for your pregnancy. I am not recommending that you restrict, or limit, your caloric intake. In fact, I'm recommending just the opposite; eat all the calories you want. Just make sure they are from the Green and Super Green food groups and the daily requirements are met. Besides, when people get hungry, they get moody. Especially pregnant women. And, if they get hungry long enough they tend to start eating whatever they can and will end up reaching out for the wrong foods.

The wrong foods not only disrupt the progress you have made, they make you gain unhealthy pregnancy weight. When you get too hungry you've most likely allowed your metabolism to become inefficient, and you are likely to start producing ketones, especially if you are pregnant. During pregnancy, when you start producing ketones your body eliminates them through the kidneys with increased urine. This can easily cause dehydration during your pregnancy, and cause you to feel even worse. Again, you should never be hungry or be lacking in food consumption with the Greens as your good guys.

Yellow Means Caution, Watch Out! The Yellow foods should be only eaten in limited amounts and cautiously. Yellow proteins include cuts of meat, poultry and dairy products that are higher in fat than Green proteins, and therefore should not be eaten in unlimited quantities. Your best choice is avoid these if at all possible. Besides, there are plenty of Green choices that are readily available.

The Yellow carbohydrates include all the starchy carbohydrates and higher fat dairy products. Starchy carbohydrates include breads, pasta, cereals, rice, and beans. The typical western diet! People in this country readily feast on a big plate of pasta for dinner, polish off a plate of pancakes for breakfast, and grab a bagel for a snack. Don't forget the biscuits at breakfast and the basket of bread with dinner. You can't go to any outdoor event without seeing something battered and fried. I'm feeling heavier just thinking about it. I understand that people have a need to eat these on occasions and will. I like to eat them on occasion too. In fact, breakfast with pancakes and bacon is my favorite meal. If you eat Yellow carbohydrates, cut back to levels that your body can handle; stay within the limits. Yellow starches can have a disastrous effect on nutrient partitioning and your metabolism. Simply put, the more Yellow carbohydrates you eat, the less fat you will burn. And, the more likely you will be to gain unhealthy weight during your pregnancy. The OB Nutritional Systems Meal Planner will tell you exactly what your Yellow carbohydrate limits are. As a side note, if you love pasta and it has been a big part of your diet, try substituting with OB Nutritional Systems Proti-pasta. It has the same taste and texture but has 20 grams of protein and is low in carbohydrates. It tastes great and you can't tell a difference except on the scales. Look for it online at **OBNutritionalSystems.com**.

Red Means Stop! Red proteins are high in fat. Red carbohydrates are highly refined, processed foods that are loaded with fructose and sugar but low in fiber. I want you to avoid Red foods as much and whenever you can. Notice I didn't say ban. I'm sure everyone has a favorite in this category and an occasional craving for it. Life wouldn't be much fun without an occasional sugar fix. You should be able to have a dessert or treat on occasion to celebrate special occasions like birthdays and anniversaries. Reaching important milestones or trimesters of your pregnancy are worth celebrating too. Hint. Hint. Otherwise, avoid them whenever you can. Just remember, if you adhere to the principles of the OB Nutritional Systems Meal Plan most of the time, you can indulge yourself on occasion without suffering the consequences.

Progressing Through the Plan

The OB Nutritional Systems Meal Plan is broken into five cycles or mini-planners. These cycles vary according to the amounts of protein, carbohydrates and fiber that you eat on a daily basis. As you progress from trimester to trimester in your pregnancy, you will start eating more Green foods, such as the lean proteins and healthy carbohydrates with high fiber. While you are increasing your Green foods you will be eating fewer Yellow foods. Yellow foods have higher fat proteins and starchy carbohydrates with low fiber. The minimum number of calories will also gradually increase as you progress from trimester to trimester. You will need to consume 150 extra calories in the second trimester and another additional 150 calories in the third trimester. The amount of protein, and the Yellow carbohydrate limit that you can consume every day depends upon your weight. The minimum amount of calories for each trimester depends on your trimester, age, height, and weight. Each OB Nutritional Systems mini planner has a chart called the OB Nutritional Systems Daily Requirements, which will tell you how many grams of protein, portions of protein, the Yellow carbohydrate limit and the amount of fiber you should consume for that cycle based upon your weight. You simply go down the weight column until you find your weight. Then scan across the columns to find the amount of proteins in grams and portions. Next, continue across to find your Yellow carbohydrate limit and the required amount of fiber in grams. You will record all these numbers and the Prenatal Calorie Need in the OB Nutritional Systems Daily Tracker. The Prenatal Calorie Need will be calculated in the OB Nutritional Systems Calorie Worksheet using information from the OB Nutritional Systems Base Calories table and the OB Nutritional Systems Height and Age Factor Calculator. I will talk about all these in detail later.

Proteins and Portions

You will notice, as you progress through the plan, that the number of grams of protein required and the number of portions of protein required gradually increases. Don't be confused by portions and grams. Since getting enough protein in your diet is key in this program, I feel it is important that you understand this completely. Getting this part down will make eating your proteins easy. Let me explain. One portion of protein equals 20 grams of protein. Three ounces of any type of meat, fish, or poultry contains about 20 grams of protein. I recommend that you get a small food scale and weigh out three ounces of each of your favorite meat, fish, and poultry choices. This will give you a quick visual reference for your portions or 20 grams. You will notice that a 3 ounce portion of these meats is roughly the size of a deck of playing cards. Therefore remember:

One Portion = 20 grams of protein = 3 ounces
(The size of a deck of playing cards)

If you will remember this relationship, you should be able to easily keep track of your protein intake. Now let's briefly talk about serving size. This is another important concept to remember. The serving size may vary and depends on how big or small the piece of meat is on your plate. The average size chicken breast is roughly the size of two decks of cards. If you served yourself one average size chicken breast that would be your serving. In this case, your serving would be the size of two decks, approximately 6 ounces, 2 portions, or 40 grams of protein. If you decided to serve yourself half of an average size chicken breast then that would be your serving. In this case your serving would be the size of 1 deck, 3 ounces, 1 portion, or 20 grams of protein. A piece of steak, also consider a serving, could be the size of four decks of cards. This would count as 4 portions or 80 g of protein. Therefore, a serving can vary in size and is used to represent the total size served. Serving size does not give you any specific size information. Therefore, your actual protein serving size per meal may equal several portions.

I will do a couple of protein samples to help illustrate. I will start with a person who weighs 140 pounds. Looking at the first trimester, OB Nutritional Systems Daily Requirements chart (page 58), I go down the weight column until I find 140 pounds. I move to the right and find 140 grams of protein is required per day, or 7 portions. This would mean I would need to eat 7 deck size portions of lean meat, poultry, or fish. If I divided up the protein requirement equally over six meals, each serving size per meal would equal roughly 1.2 portions or 23.3 grams of protein. Alternatively, or more likely, you could eat 1 portion at each of 5 meals, and then eat 2 portions at 1 meal.

Let's do one more example to make sure you got it. A 240 pound person, from the same chart, would require 240 grams of protein, or 12 portions. This would represent 12 deck size pieces of meat, or 12 portions. Divided over 6 meals, this would give a serving size per meal of 2 portions, or 40 grams of protein. Alternatively, the person might eat a large lunch of 3 portions of protein and even larger dinner of 5 portions of protein. Then, the person would only need to eat 1 portion of protein at the four other meals to meet the protein requirements. The point is, once you familiarize yourself with what a protein portion looks like, you can devise the best strategy for fulfilling your daily requirements. Make sure you understand this section completely before going on further.

It is not difficult keeping track of protein grams in dairy products. Cottage cheese is the only dairy food that provides a significant amount of protein. One cup, 8 ounces, of cottage cheese contains 30 grams of protein, or 1 ½ portions of protein. One cup is about the size of your fist if you are unable or don't want to measure it. Greek yogurt is another good source for protein with 17g of protein per 3.5 ounce serving. A slice of low-fat cheese weighs about 1 ounce and has about 7 grams of protein. One cup, 8 ounces, of nonfat yogurt contains about 10 grams of protein, or a ½ portion of protein. If you need or want the exact amounts, the number of protein grams are usually listed on packaged dairy and cheese products.

Counting Carbohydrates

The OB Nutritional Systems Food Charts (Chapter 16) has a list of common proteins and carbohydrates each subdivided into Green, Yellow, and Red categories. You will notice on the Green carbohydrates that there is no carbohydrate information. The only information listed is the fiber content. That is because you can eat as many of these as you want. You don't include them in the carbohydrate count. The Yellow carbohydrates on the other hand are more complicated. Yellow carbohydrates are found in so many shapes, sizes, and forms that their carbohydrate counts vary significantly. There is no way to uniformly measure and compare between these yellow carbohydrates. I have listed the number of carbohydrate grams for some of the more popular and common Yellow carbohydrates. For your favorites, it may be helpful to refer to the nutritional information listed on the individual product's package.

Figuring Fiber

Most fiber will come from Green carbohydrates, or from fiber supplements. The OB Nutritional Systems Food Charts provide a list of fiber content for the Green carbohydrates. The OB Nutritional Systems Daily Requirements chart will tell you how much fiber is required each day. As you become more familiar with the fiber content of your favorite foods it will be easy to quickly add them up. You will notice two cereals in the front of the Green carbohydrates section. They have a significant amount of fiber per cup. This would be an easy source to get the majority your of fiber. In fact, I eat a cup of Fiber

One every morning and eat it occasionally as a crunchy snack. That way I easily get enough fiber in my diet.

Getting It All In

The world is a hectic place. Everyone is busy, got things to do and places to be. It seems that busy schedules make eating healthy difficult. I don't have time and it is too expensive. No, it is not! Stop listening to that excuse, because it just isn't true. I find it easier, faster, and less expensive when I am eating healthy. The key is you have to plan ahead. It also helps to know where to go, what to look for if you need a serving on the run, or help meeting your requirements. I have probably already told you that I often eat on the run. I know more than half of my meals are away from the house, and I have developed a few techniques that have helped me stay on track. I have collected a few over the years from my patients. I will share all of these with you in order to make life easier for you too.

Everyone spends most of their time and focus meeting their daily protein requirement. I do it every day. I follow the maintenance phase. I weight about 140 pounds and eat about 175 grams of protein per day or approximately 9 portions. The easiest way to meet your nutritional goals is to keep things simple. Since I tend to eat the same handful of things repeatedly, keeping track is even easier. I eat the same types of protein repeatedly. I eat turkey breast, chicken breast, steak, and fish. My wife and I keep sliced turkey and chicken breast in the refrigerator all the time. We pick it up regularly from the deli, which has various types for variety. When I get hungry I reach in the refrigerator and grab a portion of meat (size of a deck of cards) and place it in a napkin and off I go. Food on the go.

We keep plenty of cans and packages of tuna fish around the house. Tuna is another open, eat and go protein portion. Dinner is most often our planned and cooked meal. Typically the core protein source will be one of the following grilled: lean beef or turkey patty, salmon, chicken breast, or steak. See, the same 5 favorite Green proteins. The variety comes in the seasonings and the assortments of Green vegetables and fruits we eat with them. Whenever we eat out, I can usually find these in a healthy selection too.

My wife keeps a variety of fresh fruits in the house for snacks. When I get in late, I often find her curled up watching television eating a bowl of watermelon. I have to fight the kids for the Cuties. We also keep protein bars, shakes, and protein powders around the house. I prefer the bars and powders for shakes. My wife prefers the readymade shakes. Whenever pasta is on the menu, we eat protein pasta which has 20 grams of protein. We keep an assortment of protein snacks around the house which include a variety of protein chips, protein wafer cookies, and chocolaty protein snacks. My favorite on the go protein sources are the protein concentrates and the ready mix drinks. You pour them into a bottled water, shake, and drink. Fifteen grams of protein, instantly. All of these protein assortments and options are available to order online at **OBNutritionalSystems.com**. If not already available, these products will soon be available at your local retail outlet.

If I find myself at a fast-food restaurant, I stick with the program. I can usually get just a plain piece of grilled chicken or a grilled chicken sandwich without the bun. I order a salad and eat the two together. If I am at a sub or wrap shop I usually fill or stuff with lots of Green proteins and Green carbohydrates. Then, I eat everything but the bread.

I make staying on track at work easy too. The first day I head to work for the week I stop off at the grocery on the way. I pick up fresh fruit and some sliced deli meat for the week. I keep protein bars and ready to mix protein smoothies at the office. I can take those with me when I leave the office heading to the hospital. I keep a couple of bottled waters in my truck and gym bag along with several packets of ready mix lemonade or fruit punch protein mix. The key is to plan ahead. It is easy to do, and you can do it too. In fact, you are probably thinking of ways to do it yourself right now. I find that my protein strategy is easy, simple, and it works for my busy schedule.

Whether you are at home or away, here are some more ideas to add protein to your diet:

- Turn a bowl of hot cereal into a high protein breakfast. Add 20 grams of unflavored protein powder to your cooked cereal. You can add fiber also.

- Turn a bowl of Fiber One cereal into a doubleheader. Add 20 grams of protein powder and now you have both protein and a great source of fiber. A real win-win.

- Super charge a serving of sugar-free or plain yogurt or low-fat cottage cheese. Add 20 grams of protein powder. You can also top off with fruit or Fiber One for extra fiber.

- Tweak unhealthy traditional pizza into a healthy protein source. Order the barbecue or grilled chicken pizza with extra chicken (my favorite) and the protein value is greatly enhanced. You can easily make your own high protein pizza at home. Take a plain ready-made pizza crust, add tomato sauce, sprinkle on low-fat mozzarella cheese, and added can of white meat chicken or grilled chicken breast. Bake until bubbly hot.

- Bump up your salad a notch or two. Add a portion or two of protein to the salad. Grilled chicken or a can of tuna will give you 20-40 grams of protein.

- Make a power omelet. Add lean ham or turkey and an assortment of green vegetables and make a good thing even better.

- Need ready on the go protein or an extra supplement. Try protein shakes, protein bars, and other protein enhanced products.

- EASY WAY TO GET PROTEIN: Get at least half of your protein from food and the rest from supplements. That is how I get my protein.

Protein shakes are an easy way to make sure that you are meeting your protein requirements for each cycle. They can be found in powder form or as prepackaged protein drinks. The prepackaged drinks can be found chilled in most convenience stores or grocery stores. Muscle milk is a common product sold. The powdered form of protein, as well as the protein drinks, is usually sold at health food stores, discount pharmacies, and supermarkets. There are two basic types of protein powders; there is the total nutrition or complete meal replacement protein. The best variety of these are made from a composite of normal milk proteins (casein and whey) and contain at least 15-30 g of protein per serving. They also have a complete array of vitamins and minerals. Meal replacements come in different flavors and can be mixed with water or low-fat or nonfat milk. Most of these products taste pretty good. The only disadvantage is they can be messy and can sometimes be difficult mixing without a blender or shaker. These products will say TOTAL NUTRITION or COMPLETE MEAL REPLACEMENT PROTEIN on the label.

The other type is the pure protein powder. Your protein powder contains protein and nothing else. A good protein powder provides up to 50 g of protein per serving. Pure protein powders are useful because they can be made into high potency protein drinks or used in cooking to enhance the protein content in meals. Pure protein powder is less expensive, but it doesn't contain the same full complement of nutrients.

Protein bars are another easy way to make sure that you meet your protein requirements. Be careful when buying protein bars because some are little more than candy bars in disguise. A high-quality protein bar should be at least 30 to 50% protein by weight. Also be aware of added sugar or high-fructose corn syrup. Some bars contain more sugar than protein. I don't recommend any protein bar which sugar or high-fructose corn syrup is listed as one of the three or four top ingredients. Quality protein bars should have twice as much protein as carbohydrates and less than 5 grams of sugar.

Some people may have difficulty getting enough daily fiber. Here are some easy ways if you are not getting enough fiber from your intake of Green carbohydrates:

- Enhance your protein shake by adding 1 cup of fresh or frozen berries.

- Use Fiber One as a substitute for breadcrumbs and croutons when cooking or fixing meals.

- Add Fiber One to your favorite cereal, sugar-free yogurt, or cottage cheese.

- Eat at least two large, mixed green salads daily. Include a mixture of high fiber vegetables.

- Add vegetables to omelets, salads and as sides to your meals.

- Use supplements such as Fibercon or sugar-free Metamucil. Remember, when you use a fiber supplement, you must be careful to drink at least two full glasses of water to avoid stomach upset.

- EASY WAY TO GET FIBER: Get at least half of your fiber from food and the rest from supplements. That is how I get my fiber.

Some people may find that suddenly increasing their fiber intake can cause gastrointestinal discomfort, such as gas and bloating. To prevent this, introduce fiber slowly and drink plenty of water. You can gradually increase your intake every day. If you have never eaten a high-fiber cereal before, start with ¼ cup and work your way up to ½ or full cup. The same is true for fruits and vegetables. If you rarely eat berries, don't start by eating 3 cups at a time. Start with a ½ cup and working your way up to more. Your body will soon get accustomed to more fiber.

A brief discussion regarding fat. There is enough fat in the food you eat. If you follow the OB Nutritional Systems Meal Plan and consume Green proteins and avoid the Yellow and Red proteins as much as possible, then you will be eating a healthy amount of fat. Be careful about added fat. We sometimes add fat to our food. Here are a few things to watch for:

- Don't add more than 1-2 tablespoons of fat to your daily diet. Fats in the form of salad dressings, butter, and other toppings and spreads.

- Order salad dressings on the side

- Cook without added fat.

- Stick to healthy fats like olive oil and omega-3 fatty acids from fish.

- Avoid trans-fatty acids. They are found in fried and processed foods and some margarine.

Finally, a short discussion on drinks. Sweetened beverages are packed with fructose and sugar. These drinks include: soda, sweet tea, fruit drinks, coffee with cream and sugar, just to name a few. They can sabotage your success on this program very quickly. Water is the drink of choice on the OB Nutritional Systems Meal Plan and the drink of choice during pregnancy too. You should drink at least eight glasses of water a day. It helps sustain a healthy hydration which helps the body promotes fat burning. Staying hydrated makes you feel better, particularly when you're pregnant. Well hydrated pregnant women are less prone to positional fainting episodes, which sometimes occurs with prolonged standing. Positional nausea is also decreased with good hydration. Real, unsweetened fruit juices are better than soda, but still not as good as whole fruit with its fiber content. It is best to try to stay away from unsweetened juices, but if you must, limit to once a week.

Milk is another source of protein, with about 8 grams protein per cup. If you drink milk, stick with the skim or 2% variety to reduce the amount of fat intake. I would limit the use of milk to coffee, cereal, and to mix with milk added protein supplements.

Coffee and tea are also ok to drink as long as you don't load them with sugar. If you must sweeten, use an artificial sweetener. Diet soda is okay if you must, but it doesn't count as water. Bubbly water, like Pierre, with a twist of lemon or lime is a better choice and it counts as water.

Best to avoid caffeine in pregnancy, but if you must, remember to limit caffeine use to no more than 1 cup of coffee, tea, soda, or other caffeinated beverage per day.

Alcohol, not while you are pregnant. Alcoholic beverages are high in sugar and carbohydrates and if you choose to have an occasional drink after your pregnancy then consume in limited quantities. However, if you really want to "lean" down, I would avoid alcohol all together.

Don't Forget Dad

I have tailored the OB Nutritional Systems Meal Plan for pregnant women, but dad can join along. In fact, I follow the maintenance phase myself along with my wife. Dad can start at the same time and phase that you start. He does not have a minimum caloric requirement like you do and therefore doesn't need to worry about calories in any of the phases. I will tell you, it helps to have a partner and definitely makes it easier when you adopt a healthy nutritional lifestyle together. Besides, you will want dad healthy and in shape to help you raise this addition to your family.

10 OB NUTRITIONAL SYSTEMS MEAL PLANNER

Let's Get Started

You are now ready to customize the OB Nutritional Systems Meal Plan to fit your pregnancy. Your planning should take into account personal food preferences and lifestyle. The meal planner will help guide you, while you create your meal plan for each trimester of your pregnancy. After the birth of your healthy baby, you will be able to plan your meals for the postpartum and recovery period. Then, once you are through the postpartum period you will be able to plan your meals and stay on a maintenance phase. This book will provide you with everything you will need to ensure your success on the meal plan. There are easy to read and easy to complete charts to help you customize the program that will best suit your needs. You can make additional copies of these charts or you can also obtain more copies online at our website **OBNutritionalSystems.com** if you prefer.

How to use the OB Nutritional Systems Meal Planner

The OB Nutritional Systems Meal Planner is divided into two parts. The first part contains the five mini-planners. The first three mini-planners are for each of the three trimesters of your pregnancy. The fourth mini-planner is for your postpartum and recovery period. The fifth and final mini-planner is for maintenance. The mini-planners each contain a quick guide, a daily requirement table, a base calorie chart, a height and age factor calculator, a calorie worksheet, a daily tracker log, a favorites list, a sample menus section, and a sample of blank menus. The second part of the OB Nutritional Systems Meal Planner is the food charts found in chapter 16, and is dedicated to outlining and organizing various foods from which you will select and use to help plan your menus for all five cycles. Within this section, you will find a set of lists that contain the Green, Yellow, and Red categories of both proteins and carbohydrates. The protein foods are broken into color categories along with their approximate calories for each 20 grams of protein. Within each color category, the proteins are divided into classes of proteins. The classes include beef, dairy, fish, game, lamb, pork, poultry, soy, and nuts. This has been done to help you find food choices faster.

The carbohydrate foods are broken into similar color categories along with their approximate calories and fiber content. Within each category the carbohydrates are also divided into classes of carbohydrates. The classes include grains, fruits, vegetables, breads and crackers, cereals, starchy vegetables, snack foods, beverages, condiments, and desserts. Again, this should help you find food items faster.

Each mini-planner starts with a description of the goals for that part of your pregnancy. It is followed by a quick guide which summarizes these goals. The description for each phase will tell you how much protein you should eat based on your current weight at the beginning of that portion of your pregnancy. The mini-planner will also tell you exactly what your Yellow carbohydrate limit will be, which is based on your current weight at the beginning of that portion of your pregnancy. The mini-planner will note the increased calorie requirement for that trimester. The minimum amount of fiber required will be the same for everyone regardless of weight.

Once you have read the goals for the trimester you're in and have a clear understanding of these goals, review them on the OB Nutritional Systems Nutritional Planner Quick Guide that follows. Then turn to the OB Nutritional Systems Daily Requirements table. This table tells you exactly how many portions of protein you should have and the number of grams of protein you should have for that phase of pregnancy. Further over on the same table, you will find the maximum allowed Yellow carbohydrates for that phase. The far right column on the table reminds you of the minimum amount of fiber in grams the phase requires. Just look up the numbers, based on your weight. The OB Nutritional Systems Calorie Worksheet along with the supporting charts will allow you to determine the minimum calories required for that trimester.

On the page that follows, you will find the OB Nutritional Systems Daily Tracker. Record your daily requirements in the top middle section below the chart's title. This helpful chart will allow you to summarize your personal daily requirements and daily achievements. This will make it easier for you to keep track of whether or not you are meeting your daily goals. Fill in your consumption of each serving by grams of protein, calories, and grams of Yellow carbohydrates for each of your six meals each day. Include along the bottom a tally of the number of grams of fiber consumed during the day. Sum up the total for each category at the end of the day to make sure that you are meeting your goals. You may find that some of you will need to do this part at the start of each trimester for only a few weeks, or until you become accustomed to your dietary needs. Others may wish to continue using the tracker for each and every week; that is fine too. The important thing is that you meet your daily goals.

The next page to follow is the OB Nutritional Systems Personal Favorites. This chart is very important, because you will find that it will be your "go to chart". You will refer to this chart several times while planning your meals because it will have the nutritional information of your most frequent choices handy. Most of us tend to eat a handful of the same foods. This habit works to our advantage by making things simple. Keeping food choices simple is the best way to succeed. Select ten of your favorite Green proteins and protein supplements and write them in the chart. If you don't have ten favorites that is okay, but list those that you do have. You can add more as you discover other favorites. Try to include at least five for both Green proteins and protein supplements. Next, list your ten favorite Green carbohydrates and Yellow carbohydrates. Again, if you don't have ten favorites list the ones that you do have. If you are short on favorites, try to come up with at least five, and you can add more as you discover them.

You will need to keep track of the following 3 numbers related to your foods. The first number is the number of calories for your favorite Green proteins, protein supplements, Green carbohydrates, and Yellow carbohydrates. This number is important to track because it will make sure you are eating enough calories. Record this number in the OB Nutritional Systems Personal Favorites chart within the calories column next to its corresponding favorite item within each listed category. The second number is the number of grams of fiber in your favorite Green carbohydrates and Yellow carbohydrates. Again, record these value in the favorites chart next to its corresponding favorite item within the listed categories. The third number is the number of carbohydrate grams in your favorite Yellow carbohydrates. This number is important to track because it will help keep you from exceeding your Yellow carbohydrate limit. Record this value in the personal favorite chart next to the corresponding favorite Yellow carbohydrate item within the listed category. Make sure to consider the actual serving size you use. For example, an item may be measured in 1 cup on the chart but you may actually use 3 cups. Make sure to account for 3 cups worth of calories, fiber and Yellow carbohydrate grams. Be sure to take in account your real portion sizes when you record the number of calories, protein, fiber, and carbohydrate grams. There is a chart for each trimester of pregnancy, the postpartum recovery period, and the maintenance phase for you to update your favorites as you transition. During pregnancy, it is common for a pregnant woman's tastes and aversions to various foods to change frequently. Keep a few extra blank copies around for each trimester in case your food cravings swing wildly, and you need to switch out and update favorites more frequently. Also, as pregnancy progresses, the caloric requirement increases slightly which might require a slight increase in portion sizes. Take the time to make any needed adjustments and complete these charts at the beginning of each trimester or sooner if needed. It will make completing your meal plans easier and make staying on track easier.

Included in the OB Nutritional Systems Meal Plan are sample menus. I intentionally kept several items non-specific. The non-specific items include fruits, vegetables, OB Nutritional Systems protein supplements, and sliced meats. For fruits, you can replace with any of the fruits in the Green carbohydrates. Keep in mind the amount of calories and fiber you need. If you need more calories and fiber then select a fruit with high calories and fiber. If you are doing well on calories and fiber then you don't have to be concerned with finding the fruits with higher counts.

For vegetables, you can replace with any of the vegetables in the Green carbohydrates. Keep in mind the amount of calories and fiber you need. If you need more calories and fiber then select a vegetable with high calories and fiber. If you are doing well on calories and fiber then you don't have to be concerned with finding the vegetables with higher counts.

The Protein supplement can be replaced with a variety of OB Nutritional Systems protein supplements or other compatible protein products, depending on availability at your leading retailer, which ever you prefer. The sliced meat you can replace with turkey or chicken slices, which ever you prefer. I will also point out, that I kept the menu to the basic and to the minimum calories and avoided the Yellow proteins and carbohydrates. This would represent the leanest and strictest menu. However, you could make it leaner if you made all the protein choices, not including protein supplements, from the Super Green proteins. The key points I want you to take out of the sample menus is how I spread out the portions and in some instances doubled them up in places. This order is not fixed you can change the order and portions around to best fit your schedule and preferences. Just make sure you at least meet the requirements for each phase. Remember, Green carbohydrates and proteins are free you can eat all you want. You could add more of these items to your menu if you wanted. Again, I was displaying the minimums. Vegetables could also mean a salad or medley. You can replace a vegetable with a mixture of vegetables, salad greens, or both. Be creative, it will add variety even in a relative small group of repetitive favorites. Notice too, the calories are omitted on the sample menus for the postpartum recovery period and the maintenance period. Since you are no longer pregnant in these phases, you do not have to be concerned about a minimum calorie intake and they are omitted.

Let's put it all together. Turn to the OB Nutritional Systems Sample Menus on page 64. Look through the sample menus and see how the food choices are laid out and organized. If you compare the items in the sample menu to the food charts starting on page 148 in chapter 16, you will see how easy it is to put simple meals together. With a little practice using the tables and food charts in the Meal Planner, you will be able to formulate your meals and create your own menus. Eventually, you will be able to track them in your head. The charts are always available just in case. You may, on occasion, discover a food item that interests you that is not listed in the chart. If this happens, the necessary information should be printed on the product box, or is included in the item's nutritional information. The information can also be easily looked up on the internet. In the search engine, type in, Nutritional information for "food name", and press enter. You will be able to quickly find the needed information. There are mobile apps available, such as Fatsecret and Fitbit, that can provide a wide range of nutritional information on various foods and food products. If you are unable to decide which category or class a food item should be placed in visit our website at **OBNutritionalSystems.com** or feel free to email me at **obnutritionalsystems@yahoo.com** and I will help you. At the end of each section you will find blank sample menus for you to fill in yourself. Make copies so you don't run out of them. You can also download more copies from our website. You are ready to get started! Turn to the corresponding mini-planner for the trimester you are in. Hopefully you started thinking about nutrition early and you are in your first trimester, if so continue reading into the next chapter.

11 FIRST TRIMESTER MINI PLANNER

OB Nutritional Systems Mini-Planner- First Trimester Goals

The first trimester of pregnancy is a busy time. A busy time for your body and metabolism! There are several changes taking place throughout the body that include physiological, emotional, and physical changes. This is mostly mediated through the changes in hormones produced while you are pregnant. Since there is so much going on inside your body, the First Trimester Mini-planner is designed to ease you into the OB Nutritional Systems program. On this program you will probably make a substantial increase in the amount of protein and fiber you consume. However, despite the saying that you are now eating for two, your calorie requirements will not change during the first trimester. Remember, the person inside is much smaller than you and does not require a lot, at least for now. You will find that you are not going to miss too many of the Yellow carbohydrates that you are accustomed to eating. Instead, we are going to let the healthy Green proteins take back their rightful place on the dinner plate, and you can send those under-minding Red carbohydrates and Red proteins packing. You will make slight changes in your eating habits. Instead of eating two or three big meals every day, and feeling starved between meals, you will start eating six mini meals throughout the day. This provides an even flow of nutrition during the day for you and your baby's needs. Eating smaller more frequent meals is actually more appetizing and helps with the nausea associated with pregnancy in most instances!

Even though these are only slight changes in eating habits, you will eventually see substantial changes in your body composition and energy levels. Over the next few weeks of your first trimester, you will notice more lean muscle than you had before. You will feel more energized and less susceptible to fatigue. Even better, you will not be storing fat or accumulating any unnecessary weight gain from your pregnancy. You will, no doubt, start mobilizing and removing some of your current fat stored for energy. This will allow you to lose unnecessary fat weight and obtain healthy weight gain in the form of muscle and weight needed for the growing pregnancy.

During the first trimester, your goal is to eat 1 gram of protein per pound of body weight daily. For example, if you weigh 125 pounds, you should eat 125 grams of protein each day. I want you to keep to the lean Green proteins and protein supplements whenever possible, for best results. As you move from the Green proteins to the Yellow and Red proteins, the amount of fat content increases and the nutritional value decreases. The more Yellow and Red proteins you consume, the more you start to increase the chance of storing fat and gaining unnecessary weight during your pregnancy. You should also limit the amount of Yellow carbohydrates you consume and stick to the Green carbohydrates as much as you can. You can use the Yellow carbohydrates to help complete your calorie count if you a short on calories after adding up your Green proteins and Green carbohydrates. If you need Yellow carbohydrates, spread them out during the day so you are not consuming them all at one setting. Do not exceed your limit on Yellow carbohydrates. In fact, you should be able to easily stay below half the Yellow limit. The calorie goal will make sure that there is plenty of calories for your daily metabolic functions including the calories needed for your developing pregnancy. You are okay if you exceed the calorie goal with Green proteins, protein supplements or Green carbohydrates. You will not gain any unnecessary weight. In fact, you can eat all of these items you want and not gain any unnecessary weight. If you do exceed the calorie goal with these foods, then make sure that you reduce, adjust, or eliminate the Yellow carbohydrates as calorie sources as indicated.

If you are currently eating the typical western diet, relatively low in protein and high in starchy Yellow carbohydrates, you will find that on OB Nutritional Systems you will be eating twice the amount of protein than you are accustomed to eating. You will also be eating leaner portions of protein as well. This should not be difficult. People generally like protein foods and are more satisfied longer when they consume them. Some people may not be able to achieve the protein quota on food alone. Protein shakes and protein bars are an easy and delicious way to get extra protein for all phases. OB Nutritional Systems does provide an assortment of delicious protein supplements including bars, shakes, smoothies, water boosters, snacks and chef sets. These are all available to order on our website at **OBNutritionalSystems.com**. The products are easy to use and convenient, whether you are at home or on the go.

Green carbohydrates are unlimited, they are all you can eat! The Green carbohydrates are also very important and it is important that you eat them frequently. Doing so, will help prevent ketosis from occurring along with its nasty side effects. Occasionally during pregnancy women have a transient ketosis, particular if they have been fasting for any length of time. Because of the frequent meals and unlimited Green Carbohydrates on the OB Nutritional Systems meal plan you should have no problem avoiding this transient condition. This unlimited amount of Green carbohydrates will allow you to increase the amount of healthy fruits and vegetables in your diet. This is a major benefit of the OB Nutritional Systems program. You will no doubt discover new favorites in the fruit and vegetable section.

I want you to restrict your Yellow carbohydrates to no more than 2 grams per pound of body weight, up to a maximum of 400 grams daily. For example, if you weigh 125 pounds, you should limit yourself to 250 grams of Yellow carbohydrates. If you weigh 225 pounds, you would limit out at 400 grams of Yellow carbohydrates. If you are following the standard western diet, this program may have less starchy carbohydrates than what you are used to eating, but it is hardly restrictive. Even if what I have recommended is less than what you normally eat, given the amount of Green protein and Green carbohydrates you will be eating, you should not feel hungry. Even though I have set a limit on the Yellow Carbohydrates, you should try to stay on the Green side of your food choices and go to the Yellow carbohydrates in a pinch. In fact you should be able to easily stay within less than half of the Yellow carbohydrate limit. Remember, more Green more lean! The leaner you are the better you will look and feel. The healthier you are the more you reduce the pregnancy risks and complications associated with poor nutrition and being overweight or obese.

During the first trimester, regardless of your weight, you need to eat at least 30 grams of fiber per day. This will most likely be more than double the amount of fiber you normally eat. I recommend eating a cup of Fiber One cereal every morning. It is listed in the Green carbohydrates and is included in the sample menus each day. This will give you approximately 28 grams of fiber for the day and will allow you to easily meet your fiber goal. You will easily get the remaining fiber from your Green carbohydrates during the day.

Now on the next few pages, take a few minutes to study and review the first trimester charts, which includes: the OB Nutritional Systems Nutrition Planner Quick Guide, the OB Nutritional Systems Daily Requirement table, the OB Nutritional Systems Base Calories table, the OB Nutritional Systems Height and Age Factor Calculator table, the OB Nutritional Systems Calorie Worksheet, and the OB Nutritional Systems Daily Tracker. Get familiar with all of these and how they interact before moving on. The quick guide gives you a brief summary of your goals for the trimester. On the daily requirements table locate your weight, and read across to determine your protein requirement and portions, yellow carbohydrate limit, and fiber requirement. Record this information in the OB Nutritional Systems Daily Tracker next to the appropriate heading.

Next you will determine the minimal calories for the first trimester. You will use the OB Nutritional Systems Base Calories first trimester table. Find your weight and move across the table to your activity level and find your base calories. Sedentary is little or no activity. Light activity is the amount of activity typically done in an office job. Moderate activity would include office work with the addition of regular exercise. Very active activity would be a job with regular and strenuous manual labor. Extra active activity requires excessive, frequent, and intense physical activity, such as the type of activity performed by professional athletes during intense training. Enter your base calories in the OB Nutritional Systems Calorie Worksheet on the line provided next to Base Calories. Next, use the OB Nutritional Systems Height and Age Factor Calculator chart to locate your height and age factors. Find your height and move across to your height factor and record this number in the line provided next to Height Factor in the OB Nutritional Systems Calorie Worksheet. Find your age and move across to your age factor and record this number in the line provided next to Age Factor in the OB Nutritional Systems Calorie Worksheet. Calculate your Prenatal Caloric Need by adding together the Base Calories, Height Factor, and Age Factor. Record the total on the space provided on the worksheet and record in the appropriate place in the OB Nutritional Systems Daily Tracker First Trimester.

You can then use the daily tracker to record your daily intake at each meal of your proteins, calories and yellow carbohydrates to help you make sure you are following the requirements. You will soon be able to keep track of everything in your head once you become familiar with the process. Afterward, look at the food items in chapter 16, starting on page 148, and find your favorites and record them on the OB Nutritional Systems Personal Favorites chart. Then, using your favorites chart, sample menus, and blank menus create your own menu plans. Again, once you get familiar with the system you will be able to do all this in your head. When you are able to follow the system in your head, you will begin creating a nutritious habit and be on your way to adopting a healthy nutritional lifestyle. Remember to keep it simple and have fun planning.

OB NUTRITIONAL SYSTEMS NUTRITION PLANNER QUICK GUIDE

------ **FIRST TRIMESTER** ------

Nutrient	
Protein	1 gram per pound of body weight Green protein: Your protein choices should come from these foods. Yellow protein: Avoid if possible but no more than 2 servings from this group per week. Red protein: Avoid. Special occasions only.
Carbohydrates	2 gram per pound of body weight. (Up to maximum of 400g yellow carbohydrates per day.) Green carbohydrates: Unlimited, does not count toward your total. Yellow carbohydrates: Caution with these, stick within the limits. Red carbohydrates: Avoid. Special occasions only and count toward limit.
Fiber	30 grams
Prenatal Caloric Need	Base Calories First Trimester + Age Factor + Height Factor

OB NUTRITIONAL SYSTEMS DAILY REQUIREMENTS
FIRST TRIMESTER

Enter information for your weight in the OB Nutritional Systems Daily Tracker First Trimester

3 ounces of protein = 20 usable grams of protein = 1 serving

(roughyl the size of a deck of playing cards)

Weight	Protein Grams	Protein Portions	Yellow Carb Limit Grams	Fiber Grams
70	70	4	140	30
80	80	4	160	30
90	90	5	180	30
100	100	5	200	30
110	110	6	220	30
120	120	6	240	30
130	130	7	260	30
140	140	7	280	30
150	150	8	300	30
160	160	8	320	30
170	170	9	340	30
180	180	9	360	30
190	190	10	380	30
200	200	10	400	30
210	210	11	400	30
220	220	11	400	30
230	230	12	400	30
240	240	12	400	30
250	250	13	400	30
260	260	13	400	30
270	270	14	400	30
280	280	14	400	30
290	290	15	400	30
300	300	15	400	30
310	310	16	400	30
320	320	16	400	30
330	330	17	400	30
340	340	17	400	30
350	350	18	400	30
360	360	18	400	30

OB NUTRITIONAL SYSTEMS BASE CALORIES
FIRST TRIMESTER

Enter the base calories for your weight and activity level in the OB Nutritional Systems
Calorie Worksheet First Trimester.

Weight	Sedentary	Lightly Active	Moderately Active	Very Active	Extra Active
70	786	900	1015	1129	1244
80	841	963	1086	1208	1330
90	895	1025	1156	1286	1417
100	950	1088	1227	1365	1503
110	1004	1150	1297	1443	1590
120	1059	1213	1368	1522	1676
130	1114	1275	1438	1600	1763
140	1168	1338	1509	1679	1849
150	1223	1401	1579	1757	1936
160	1278	1463	1650	1836	2022
170	1332	1526	1721	1914	2109
180	1387	1588	1791	1993	2195
190	1441	1651	1862	2071	2282
200	1496	1714	1932	2150	2368
210	1551	1776	2003	2228	2455
220	1605	1839	2073	2307	2541
230	1660	1901	2144	2385	2628
240	1715	1964	2214	2464	2714
250	1769	2026	2285	2542	2801
260	1824	2089	2355	2621	2887
270	1878	2152	2426	2699	2974
280	1933	2214	2497	2778	3060
290	1988	2277	2567	2856	3147
300	2042	2339	2638	2935	3233
310	2097	2402	2708	3013	3320
320	2152	2465	2779	3092	3406
330	2206	2527	2849	3170	3492
340	2261	2590	2920	3249	3579
350	2315	2652	2990	3327	3665
360	2370	2715	3061	3406	3752

OB NUTRITIONAL SYSTEMS HEIGHT AND AGE FACTOR CALCULATOR

Enter the height and age factors for your height and age in the OB Nutritional Systems Calorie Worksheet First Trimester

Height	Height Factor	Age	Age Factor
4'0"	0	50	0
4'1"	22	49	6
4'2"	44	48	12
4'3"	66	47	18
4'4"	88	46	24
4'5"	110	45	30
4'6"	132	44	36
4'7"	154	43	42
4'8"	176	42	48
4'9"	198	41	54
4'10"	220	40	60
4'11"	242	39	66
5'0"	264	38	72
5'1"	286	37	78
5'2"	308	36	84
5'3"	330	35	90
5'4"	352	34	96
5'5"	374	33	102
5'6"	396	32	108
5'7"	418	31	114
5'8"	440	30	120
5'9"	462	29	126
5'10"	484	28	132
5'11"	506	27	138
6'0"	528	26	144
6'1"	550	25	150
6'2"	572	24	156
6'3"	594	23	162
6'4"	616	22	168
6'5"	638	21	174
6'6"	660	20	180
6'7"	682	19	186
6'8"	704	18	192
6'9"	726	17	198
6'10"	748	16	204
6'11"	770	15	210
7'0"	792	14	216
7'1"	814	13	222
7'2"	836	12	228

OB NUTRITIONAL SYSTEMS CALORIE WORKSHEET

------ FIRST TRIMESTER ------

Enter the Base Calories for your weight and activity level from the OB Nutritional Systems Base Calories First Trimester table.	**Base Calories =** _____
Enter Height Factor for your height from the OB Nutritional Systems Height and Age Calculator.	**Height Factor =** _____
Enter Age Factor for your age from the OB Nutritional Systems Height and Age Calculator.	**Age Factor =** _____
Calculate **Prenatal Caloric Need**: Start with **Base Calories** and add the **Height Factor** and then add the **Age** and then enter the total as the **Prenatal Caloric Need**.	**Prenatal Caloric Need =** _____ Enter this number in the calorie goal on the OB Nutritional Systems Daily Tracker-First Trimester.

OB NUTRITIONAL SYSTEMS DAILY TRACKER
YOUR DAILY REQUIRMENTS
FIRST TRIMESTER

Protein goal in grams: _____

Protein goal in servings: _____

Prenatal Caloric Need: _____

Yellow Carbohydrate limit in grams: _____

Fiber goal in grams: _____

Meals

		1	2	3	4	5	6	Totals	Total fiber
Day 1	Protein								
	Calorie								
	Carbs								
Day 2	Protein								
	Calorie								
	Carbs								
Day 3	Protein								
	Calorie								
	Carbs								
Day 4	Protein								
	Calorie								
	Carbs								
Day 5	Protein								
	Calorie								
	Carbs								
Day 6	Protein								
	Calorie								
	Carbs								
Day 7	Protein								
	Calorie								
	Carbs								

OB NUTRITIONAL SYSTEMS PERSONAL FAVORITES
FIRST TRIMESTER

Green Protein	Calories	Grams Protein	Green Carbohydrates	Calories	Grams Fiber	
1			1			
2			2			
3			3			
4			4			
5			5			
6			6			
7			7			
8			8			
9			9			
10			10			

Protein Supplement	Calories	Grams Protein	Yellow Carbohydrates	Calories	Grams Fiber	Grams Carbs
1			1			
2			2			
3			3			
4			4			
5			5			
6			6			
7			7			
8			8			
9			9			
10			10			

Select your 10 favorite Green Proteins, Protein Supplements, Green Carbohydrates, and Yellow Carbohydrates. You can plan most of your meals with these. Keep track of calories on all items. Keep track of grams of protein for Green Protein and Protein Supplements. Keep track of grams of carbs on the Yellow Carbohydrates. (Don't Exceed Limit)

OB NUTRITIONAL SYSTEMS SAMPLE MENUS
FIRST TRIMESTER: 35 y/o, 5'4", 150 pound Sedentary Woman
DAY 1

MEAL	DESCRIPTION
1.	1. Eggs (3) 1 portion = 20 grams protein and 270 calories. 2. Vegetable serving = 75 calories and 3 grams fiber. 3. Fruit serving = 75 calories and 3 grams fiber.
2.	1. OBNS Protein Supplement 1 portion = 15 grams protein, 160 calories, and 3 grams fiber. 2. Fruit serving = 75 calories and 3 grams fiber.
3.	1. Sliced meat 2 portions =40g protein and 200 calories. 2. Vegetables 2 servings = 150 calories and 6 grams fiber. 3. Fruit serving = 75 calories and 3 grams fiber.
4.	1. OBNS Protein Supplement 1 portion =20 grams protein, 110 calories and 3 grams fiber. 2. Fruit serving = 75 calories and 3 grams fiber.
5.	1. Grilled Salmon 2 portions = 40 grams protein and 200 calories. 2. Vegetables 2 servings = 150 calories and 6 grams fiber. 3. Fruit 2 servings = 150 calories, 6 grams of fiber.
6.	1. Sliced meat 1 portion =20 grams protein and 100 calories. 2. Fruit serving = 75 calories and 3 grams fiber **Totals: Protein 150 grams in 8 portions, Calories 1940, fiber 42 grams, Yellow carbs 0 grams**

DAY 2

MEAL	DESCRIPTION
1.	1. OBNS Protein Supplement 1 portion = 20 grams protein, 110 calories, and 5 grams fiber 2. Vegetable serving = 75 calories and 3 grams fiber. 3. Fruit 2 servings = 150 calories and 6 grams fiber.
2.	1. OBNS Protein Supplement 1 portion = 15 grams protein, 160 calories, and 3 grams fiber. 2. Fruit 2 servings = 150 calories and 6 grams fiber.
3.	1. Sliced meat 2 portions =40g protein and 200 calories. 2. Vegetables 2 servings = 150 calories and 6 grams fiber. 3. Fruit serving = 75 calories and 3 grams fiber.
4.	1. OBNS Protein Supplement 1 portion =20 grams protein, 110 calories and 3 grams fiber. 2. Fruit serving = 75 calories and 3 grams fiber.
5.	1. Grilled Chicken 2 portions = 40 grams protein and 200 calories. 2. Vegetables 2 servings = 150 calories and 6 grams fiber. 3. Fruit 2 servings = 150 calories, 6 grams of fiber.
6.	1. Sliced meat 1 portion =20 grams protein and 100 calories. 2. Fruit 1 serving = 75 calories and 3 grams fiber **Totals: Protein 150 grams in 8 portions, Calories 1930, fiber 53 grams, Yellow carbs 0 grams**

OB NUTRITIONAL SYSTEMS SAMPLE MENUS
FIRST TRIMESTER: 35 y/o, 5'4", 150 pound Sedentary Woman
DAY 3

MEAL	DESCRIPTION
1.	1. Eggs (3) 1 portion = 20 grams protein and 270 calories. 2. Vegetable serving = 75 calories and 3 grams fiber. 3. Fruit serving = 75 calories and 3 grams fiber.
2.	1. OBNS Protein Supplement 1 portion = 15 grams protein, 160 calories, and 3 grams fiber. 2. Fruit serving = 75 calories and 3 grams fiber.
3.	1. Tuna 2 portions =40g protein and 200 calories. 2. Vegetables 2 servings = 150 calories and 6 grams fiber. 3. Fruit serving = 75 calories and 3 grams fiber.
4.	1. OBNS Protein Supplement 1 portion =20 grams protein, 110 calories and 3 grams fiber. 2. Fruit serving = 75 calories and 3 grams fiber.
5.	1. Lean burger patties 2 portions = 40 grams protein and 200 calories. 2. Vegetables 2 servings = 150 calories and 6 grams fiber. 3. Fruit 2 servings = 150 calories, 6 grams of fiber.
6.	1. Sliced meat 1 portion =20 grams protein and 100 calories. 2. Fruit serving = 75 calories and 3 grams fiber **Totals: Protein 150 grams in 8 portions, Calories 1940, fiber 42 grams, Yellow carbs 0 grams**

DAY 4

MEAL	DESCRIPTION
1.	1. Eggs (3) 1 portion = 20 grams protein and 270 calories. 2. Vegetable serving = 75 calories and 3 grams fiber. 3. Fruit serving = 75 calories and 3 grams fiber.
2.	1. OBNS Protein Supplement 1 portion = 15 grams protein, 160 calories, and 3 grams fiber. 2. Fruit serving = 75 calories and 3 grams fiber.
3.	1. Sliced meat 2 portions =40g protein and 200 calories. 2. Vegetables 2 servings = 150 calories and 6 grams fiber. 3. Fruit serving = 75 calories and 3 grams fiber.
4.	1. OBNS Protein Supplement 1 portion =20 grams protein, 110 calories and 3 grams fiber. 2. Fruit serving = 75 calories and 3 grams fiber.
5.	1. Grilled Chicken 2 portions = 40 grams protein and 200 calories. 2. Vegetables 2 servings = 150 calories and 6 grams fiber. 3. Fruit 2 servings = 150 calories, 6 grams of fiber.
6.	1. Sliced meat 1 portion =20 grams protein and 100 calories. 2. Fruit serving = 75 calories and 3 grams fiber **Totals: Protein 150 grams in 8 portions, Calories 1940, fiber 42 grams, Yellow carbs 0 grams**

OB NUTRITIONAL SYSTEMS SAMPLE MENUS
FIRST TRIMESTER: 35 y/o, 5'4", 150 pound Sedentary Woman
DAY 5

MEAL	DESCRIPTION
1.	1. Eggs (3) 1 portion = 20 grams protein and 270 calories. 2. Vegetable serving = 75 calories and 3 grams fiber. 3. Fruit serving = 75 calories and 3 grams fiber.
2.	1. OBNS Protein Supplement 1 portion = 15 grams protein, 160 calories, and 3 grams fiber. 2. Fruit serving = 75 calories and 3 grams fiber.
3.	1. Sliced meat 2 portions =40g protein and 200 calories. 2. Vegetables 2 servings = 150 calories and 6 grams fiber. 3. Fruit serving = 75 calories and 3 grams fiber.
4.	1. OBNS Protein Supplement 1 portion =20 grams protein, 110 calories and 3 grams fiber. 2. Fruit serving = 75 calories and 3 grams fiber.
5.	1. Protein Pasta with lean meat sauce 2 portions = 40 grams protein and 200 calories. 2. Vegetables 2 servings = 150 calories and 6 grams fiber. 3. Fruit 2 servings = 150 calories, 6 grams of fiber.
6.	1. Sliced meat 1 portion =20 grams protein and 100 calories. 2. Fruit serving = 75 calories and 3 grams fiber

Totals: Protein 150 grams in 8 portions, Calories 1940, fiber 42 grams, Yellow carbs 0 grams

DAY 6

MEAL	DESCRIPTION
1.	1. OBNS Protein Supplement 1 portion = 20 grams protein, 110 calories, and 5 grams fiber 2. Vegetable serving = 75 calories and 3 grams fiber. 3. Fruit 2 servings = 150 calories and 6 grams fiber.
2.	1. OBNS Protein Supplement 1 portion = 15 grams protein, 160 calories, and 3 grams fiber. 2. Fruit serving = 75 calories and 3 grams fiber.
3.	1. Sliced meat 2 portions =40g protein and 200 calories. 2. Vegetables 2 servings = 150 calories and 6 grams fiber. 3. Fruit serving = 75 calories and 3 grams fiber.
4.	1. OBNS Protein Supplement 1 portion =20 grams protein, 110 calories and 3 grams fiber. 2. Fruit serving = 75 calories and 3 grams fiber.
5.	1. Grilled Salmon 2 portions = 40 grams protein and 200 calories. 2. Vegetables 2 servings = 150 calories and 6 grams fiber. 3. Fruit 2 servings = 150 calories, 6 grams of fiber.
6.	1. Sliced meat 1 portion =20 grams protein and 100 calories. 2. Fruit 2 servings = 150 calories and 6 grams fiber

Totals: Protein 150 grams in 8 portions, Calories 1930, fiber 53 grams, Yellow carbs 0 grams

OB NUTRITIONAL SYSTEMS SAMPLE MENUS
FIRST TRIMESTER: 35 y/o, 5'4", 150 pound Sedentary Woman
DAY 7

MEAL	DESCRIPTION
1.	1. OBNS Protein Supplement 1 portion = 20 grams protein, 110 calories, and 5 grams fiber 2. Vegetable serving = 75 calories and 3 grams fiber. 3. Fruit 2 servings = 150 calories and 6 grams fiber.
2.	1. OBNS Protein Supplement 1 portion = 15 grams protein, 160 calories, and 3 grams fiber. 2. Fruit serving = 75 calories and 3 grams fiber.
3.	1. Sliced meat 2 portions =40g protein and 200 calories. 2. Vegetables 2 servings = 150 calories and 6 grams fiber. 3. Fruit serving = 75 calories and 3 grams fiber.
4.	1. OBNS Protein Supplement 1 portion =20 grams protein, 110 calories and 3 grams fiber. 2. Fruit serving = 75 calories and 3 grams fiber.
5.	1. Steak 2 portions = 40 grams protein and 400 calories. 2. Vegetables 2 servings = 150 calories and 6 grams fiber. 3. Fruit 1 servings = 75 calories, 3 grams of fiber.
6.	1. Sliced meat 1 portion =20 grams protein and 100 calories. 2. 1 Fruit serving = 75 calories and 3 grams fiber **Totals: Protein 150 grams in 8 portions, Calories 1980, fiber 47 grams, Yellow carbs 0 grams**

BLANK MENUS
FIRST TRIMESTER
DAY 1

MEAL	DESCRIPTION
1.	
2.	
3.	
4.	
5.	
6.	

BLANK MENUS
FIRST TRIMESTER
DAY 2

MEAL	DESCRIPTION
1.	
2.	
3.	
4.	
5.	
6.	

BLANK MENUS
FIRST TRIMESTER
DAY 3

MEAL	DESCRIPTION
1.	
2.	
3.	
4.	
5.	
6.	

BLANK MENUS
FIRST TRIMESTER
DAY 4

MEAL	DESCRIPTION
1.	
2.	
3.	
4.	
5.	
6.	

BLANK MENUS
FIRST TRIMESTER
DAY 5

MEAL	DESCRIPTION
1.	
2.	
3.	
4.	
5.	
6.	

BLANK MENUS
FIRST TRIMESTER
DAY 6

MEAL	DESCRIPTION
1.	
2.	
3.	
4.	
5.	
6.	

BLANK MENUS
FIRST TRIMESTER
DAY 7

MEAL	DESCRIPTION
1.	
2.	
3.	
4.	
5.	
6.	

12 SECOND TRIMESTER MINI PLANNER

OB Nutritional Systems Mini-Planner-Second Trimester Goals

During the second trimester you will start to notice the increase in physical demands on your body as a result of the pregnancy. However, you have been preparing for this increase demand during the last trimester by eating healthy and building lean muscle. You should be able to take this trimester in stride. During this time you will start to notice movement from your baby. A time of great satisfaction and a time when the pregnancy starts to really feel real! If you were fortunate to have started with us during your first trimester, then you should be feeling good about yourself and your pregnancy. For most, the nausea has subsided. You should be feeling the benefits of healthy nutrition. You will have avoided gaining any unnecessary weight from fat. You should notice an increase in your lean muscle. All of which should make you feel stronger and healthier.

If you are just now joining us, I recommend starting with the first trimester program. Then, after an abbreviated course of 4 to 6 weeks, move up to join the last half of the second trimester program. Also, if you have been with the program and you are still feeling a little overwhelmed with the transition, or need more time to transition, that is completely understandable. You also can continue with the first trimester mini-planner. Whichever circumstance, if you choose to continue with the first trimester mini-planner you still have to increase your calories by 150 calories during the second trimester and another 150 calories in the third trimester. That is the only adjustment that you will have to make. You can get those extra calories from your Green carbohydrates.

Moving on. In the second trimester you will increase your protein intake to 1.25 grams of protein per pound of body weight per day. This means you will have an additional serving or two of protein per day. Make most of your selections from the lean, Green protein list or from protein supplements. Continue to avoid the Yellow and Red proteins. Limited any Yellow proteins to one serving a week.

In the second trimester you will also increase the minimum number of calories by a 150 calories per day. This is roughly the equivalent of two servings of fresh fruit or 5 graham crackers per day. This will be enough additional calories to meet the increased metabolic demands of the pregnancy and your growing baby.

The Green carbohydrates continue to be unlimited, so enjoy them. They are free! You will reduce your Yellow carbohydrate intake to 1 gram per pound of body weight during the second trimester. A maximum of 400 grams per day if you weigh over 400 pounds. You should not feel deprived of Yellow carbohydrates, because most people, by this point, are eating less than this limit all ready.

During the second trimester you will increase the minimum fiber intake to 40 grams. Again, if you are including a daily bowl of Fiber One cereal in your meal plan, then you are most likely already meeting this goal.

Now, review the OB Nutritional Systems Quick Guide and Daily Requirement pages for the second trimester to determine the protein, portion, and fiber requirements, and the yellow carbohydrate limit for your second trimester. Review the OB Nutritional Systems Base Calories for the second trimester along with the Height and Age Factor Calculator chart to obtain the values to include in the OB Nutritional Systems Calorie Worksheet for the second trimester. Add those numbers together to get your second trimester Prenatal Caloric Need. Then, use all the information to complete the daily requirements in your OB Nutritional Systems Daily Tracker. Afterward, update your favorites on the OB Nutritional Systems Personal Favorites chart. Again, using the sample menus, use your favorites list and other food items from the table to create your menus. Remember to keep it simple.

OB NUTRITIONAL SYSTEMS NUTRITION PLANNER QUICK GUIDE

------ SECOND TRIMESTER ------

Nutrient	
Protein	1.25 grams per pound of body weight Green protein: Your protein choices should come from these foods. Yellow protein: Avoid if possible but limited to 1 serving per week. Red protein: Avoid. Special occasions only.
Carbohydrates	1 gram per pound of body weight. (Up to maximum of 400g yellow carbohydrates per day.) Green carbohydrates: Unlimited, does not count toward your total. Yellow carbohydrates: Caution with these, stick within the limits. Red carbohydrates: Avoid. Special occasions only and count toward limit.
Fiber	40 grams
Prenatal Caloric Need	Base Calories Second Trimester + Age Factor + Height Factor

OB NUTRITIONAL SYSTEMS DAILY REQUIREMENTS
SECOND TRIMESTER
Enter information for your weight in the OB Nutritional Systems Daily Tracker Second Trimester

3 ounces of protein = 20 usable grams of protein = 1 serving

(roughyl the size of a deck of playing cards)

Weight	Protein Grams	Protein Portions	Yellow Carb Limit Grams	Fiber Grams
70	88	4	70	40
80	100	5	80	40
90	113	6	90	40
100	125	6	100	40
110	138	7	110	40
120	150	8	120	40
130	163	8	130	40
140	175	9	140	40
150	188	9	150	40
160	200	10	160	40
170	213	11	170	40
180	225	11	180	40
190	238	12	190	40
200	250	13	200	40
210	263	13	210	40
220	275	14	220	40
230	288	14	230	40
240	300	15	240	40
250	313	16	250	40
260	325	16	260	40
270	338	17	270	40
280	350	18	280	40
290	363	18	290	40
300	375	19	300	40
310	388	19	310	40
320	400	20	320	40
330	413	21	330	40
340	425	21	340	40
350	438	22	350	40
360	450	23	360	40

OB NUTRITIONAL SYSTEMS BASE CALORIES
SECOND TRIMESTER

Enter the base calories for your weight and activity level in the OB Nutritional Systems Calorie Worksheet Second Trimester.

Weight	Sedentary	Lightly Active	Moderately Active	Very Active	Extra Active
70	936	1050	1165	1279	1394
80	991	1113	1236	1358	1480
90	1045	1175	1306	1436	1567
100	1100	1238	1377	1515	1653
110	1154	1300	1447	1593	1740
120	1209	1363	1518	1672	1826
130	1264	1425	1588	1750	1913
140	1318	1488	1659	1829	1999
150	1373	1551	1729	1907	2086
160	1428	1613	1800	1986	2172
170	1482	1676	1871	2064	2259
180	1537	1738	1941	2143	2345
190	1591	1801	2012	2221	2432
200	1646	1864	2082	2300	2518
210	1701	1926	2153	2378	2605
220	1755	1989	2223	2457	2691
230	1810	2051	2294	2535	2778
240	1865	2114	2364	2614	2864
250	1919	2176	2435	2692	2951
260	1974	2239	2505	2771	3037
270	2028	2302	2576	2849	3124
280	2083	2364	2647	2928	3210
290	2138	2427	2717	3006	3297
300	2192	2489	2788	3085	3383
310	2247	2552	2858	3163	3470
320	2302	2615	2929	3242	3556
330	2356	2677	2999	3320	3642
340	2411	2740	3070	3399	3729
350	2465	2802	3140	3477	3815
360	2520	2865	3211	3556	3902

OB NUTRITIONAL SYSTEMS HEIGHT AND AGE FACTOR CALCULATOR

Enter the height and age factors for your height and age in the OB Nutritional Systems
Calorie Worksheet Second Trimester

Height	Height Factor		Age	Age Factor
4'0"	0		50	0
4'1"	22		49	6
4'2"	44		48	12
4'3"	66		47	18
4'4"	88		46	24
4'5"	110		45	30
4'6"	132		44	36
4'7"	154		43	42
4'8"	176		42	48
4'9"	198		41	54
4'10"	220		40	60
4'11"	242		39	66
5'0"	264		38	72
5'1"	286		37	78
5'2"	308		36	84
5'3"	330		35	90
5'4"	352		34	96
5'5"	374		33	102
5'6"	396		32	108
5'7"	418		31	114
5'8"	440		30	120
5'9"	462		29	126
5'10"	484		28	132
5'11"	506		27	138
6'0"	528		26	144
6'1"	550		25	150
6'2"	572		24	156
6'3"	594		23	162
6'4"	616		22	168
6'5"	638		21	174
6'6"	660		20	180
6'7"	682		19	186
6'8"	704		18	192
6'9"	726		17	198
6'10"	748		16	204
6'11"	770		15	210
7'0"	792		14	216
7'1"	814		13	222
7'2"	836		12	228

OB NUTRITIONAL SYSTEMS CALORIE WORKSHEET

------ SECOND TRIMESTER ------

Enter the Base Calories for your weight and activity level from the OB Nutritional Systems Base Calories Second Trimester table.	**Base Calories =** _____
Enter Height Factor for your height from the OB Nutritional Systems Height and Age Calculator.	**Height Factor =** _____
Enter Age Factor for your age from the OB Nutritional Systems Height and Age Calculator.	**Age Factor =** _____
Calculate **Prenatal Caloric Need**: Start with **Base Calories** and add the **Height Factor** and then add the **Age** and then enter the total as the **Prenatal Caloric Need**.	**Prenatal Caloric Need =** _____ Enter this number in the calorie goal on the OB Nutritional Systems Daily Tracker-Second Trimester.

OB NUTRITIONAL SYSTEMS DAILY TRACKER
YOUR DAILY REQUIRMENTS
SECOND TRIMESTER

Protein goal in grams: _____

Protein goal in servings: _____

Prenatal Caloric Need: _____

Yellow Carbohydrate limit in grams: _____

Fiber goal in grams: _____

		Meals 1	2	3	4	5	6	Totals	Total fiber
Day 1	Protein								
	Calorie								
	Carbs								
Day 2	Protein								
	Calorie								
	Carbs								
Day 3	Protein								
	Calorie								
	Carbs								
Day 4	Protein								
	Calorie								
	Carbs								
Day 5	Protein								
	Calorie								
	Carbs								
Day 6	Protein								
	Calorie								
	Carbs								
Day 7	Protein								
	Calorie								
	Carbs								

OB NUTRITIONAL SYSTEMS PERSONAL FAVORITES
SECOND TRIMESTER

Green Protein	Calories	Grams Protein	Green Carbohydrates	Calories	Grams Fiber
1			1		
2			2		
3			3		
4			4		
5			5		
6			6		
7			7		
8			8		
9			9		
10			10		

Protein Supplement	Calories	Grams Protein	Yellow Carbohydrates	Calories	Grams Fiber	Grams Carbs
1			1			
2			2			
3			3			
4			4			
5			5			
6			6			
7			7			
8			8			
9			9			
10			10			

Select your 10 favorite Green Proteins, Protein Supplements, Green Carbohydrates, and Yellow Carbohydrates. You can plan most of your meals with these. Keep track of calories on all items. Keep track of grams of protein for Green Protein and Protein Supplements. Keep track of grams of carbs on the Yellow Carbohydrates. (Don't Exceed Limit)

OB NUTRITIONAL SYSTEMS SAMPLE MENUS
SECOND TRIMESTER: 35 y/o, 5'4", 150 pound Sedentary Woman
DAY 1

MEAL	DESCRIPTION
1.	1. Eggs (3) 1 portion = 20 grams protein and 270 calories. 2. Vegetable serving = 75 calories and 6 grams fiber. 3. Fruit serving = 75 calories and 3 grams fiber.
2.	1. OBNS Protein Supplement 1 portion = 15 grams protein, 160 calories, and 3 grams fiber. 2. Fruit serving = 75 calories and 3 grams fiber. 3. Sliced meat 1 portion = 20 grams protein and 100 calories.
3.	1. Sliced meat 2 portions =40g protein and 200 calories. 2. Vegetables 2 servings = 150 calories and 12 grams fiber. 3. Fruit serving = 75 calories and 3 grams fiber.
4.	1. OBNS Protein Supplement 1 portion =20 grams protein, 110 calories and 3 grams fiber. 2. Fruit serving = 75 calories and 3 grams fiber.
5.	1. Grilled Salmon 2 portions = 40 grams protein and 200 calories. 2. Vegetables 2 servings = 150 calories and 6 grams fiber. 3. Fruit 1 servings = 75 calories, 3 grams of fiber.
6.	1. Sliced meat 2 portion =40 grams protein and 200 calories. 2. Fruit serving = 75 calories and 3 grams fiber **Totals: Protein 190 grams in 10 portions, Calories 2065, fiber 46 grams, Yellow carbs 0 grams**

DAY 2

MEAL	DESCRIPTION
1.	1. OBNS Protein Supplement 1 portion = 20 grams protein, 110 calories, and 5 grams fiber 2. Vegetable serving = 75 calories and 3 grams fiber. 3. Fruit 2 servings = 150 calories and 6 grams fiber.
2.	1. OBNS Protein Supplement 1 portion = 15 grams protein, 160 calories, and 3 grams fiber. 2. Fruit 1 servings = 75 calories and 6 grams fiber. 3. Sliced meat 1 portion = 20 grams protein and 100 calories.
3.	1. Sliced meat 2 portions =40g protein and 200 calories. 2. Vegetables 2 servings = 150 calories and 6 grams fiber. 3. Fruit serving = 75 calories and 3 grams fiber.
4.	1. OBNS Protein Supplement 1 portion =20 grams protein, 110 calories and 3 grams fiber. 2. Fruit serving = 75 calories and 3 grams fiber.
5.	1. Grilled Chicken 2 portions = 40 grams protein and 200 calories. 2. Vegetables 2 servings = 150 calories and 6 grams fiber. 3. Fruit 2 servings = 150 calories, 6 grams of fiber.
6.	1. Sliced meat 2 portion =40 grams protein and 200 calories. 2. Fruit 1 serving = 75 calories and 3 grams fiber **Totals: Protein 190 grams in 10 portions, Calories 2065, fiber 53 grams, Yellow carbs 0 grams**

OB NUTRITIONAL SYSTEMS SAMPLE MENUS
SECOND TRIMESTER: 35 y/o, 5'4", 150 pound Sedentary Woman
DAY 3

MEAL	DESCRIPTION
1.	1. Eggs (3) 1 portion = 20 grams protein and 270 calories. 2. Vegetable serving = 75 calories and 6 grams fiber. 3. Fruit serving = 75 calories and 3 grams fiber.
2.	1. OBNS Protein Supplement 1 portion = 15 grams protein, 160 calories, and 3 grams fiber. 2. Fruit serving = 75 calories and 3 grams fiber. 3. Sliced meat 1 portion = 20 grams protein and 100 calories.
3.	1. Tuna 2 portions =40g protein and 200 calories. 2. Vegetables 2 servings = 150 calories and 6 grams fiber. 3. Fruit serving = 75 calories and 3 grams fiber.
4.	1. OBNS Protein Supplement 1 portion =20 grams protein, 110 calories and 3 grams fiber. 2. Fruit serving = 75 calories and 3 grams fiber.
5.	1. Lean burger patties 2 portions = 40 grams protein and 200 calories. 2. Vegetables 2 servings = 150 calories and 6 grams fiber. 3. Fruit 1 servings = 75 calories, 6 grams of fiber.
6.	1. Sliced meat 2 portion =40 grams protein and 200 calories. 2. Fruit serving = 75 calories and 3 grams fiber **Totals: Protein 190 grams in 10 portions, Calories 2065, fiber 45 grams, Yellow carbs 0 grams**

DAY 4

MEAL	DESCRIPTION
1.	1. Eggs (3) 1 portion = 20 grams protein and 270 calories. 2. Vegetable serving = 75 calories and 6 grams fiber. 3. Fruit serving = 75 calories and 3 grams fiber.
2.	1. OBNS Protein Supplement 1 portion = 15 grams protein, 160 calories, and 3 grams fiber. 2. Fruit serving = 75 calories and 3 grams fiber. 3. Sliced meat 1 portion = 20 grams protein and 100 calories.
3.	1. Sliced meat 2 portions =40g protein and 200 calories. 2. Vegetables 2 servings = 150 calories and 6 grams fiber. 3. Fruit serving = 75 calories and 3 grams fiber.
4.	1. OBNS Protein Supplement 1 portion =20 grams protein, 110 calories and 3 grams fiber. 2. Fruit serving = 75 calories and 3 grams fiber.
5.	1. Grilled Chicken 2 portions = 40 grams protein and 200 calories. 2. Vegetables 2 servings = 150 calories and 6 grams fiber. 3. Fruit 1 servings = 75 calories, 6 grams of fiber.
6.	1. Sliced meat 2 portion =40 grams protein and 200 calories. 2. Fruit serving = 75 calories and 3 grams fiber **Totals: Protein 190 grams in 10 portions, Calories 2065, fiber 45 grams, Yellow carbs 0 grams**

OB NUTRITIONAL SYSTEMS SAMPLE MENUS
SECOND TRIMESTER: 35 y/o, 5'4", 150 pound Sedentary Woman
DAY 5

MEAL	DESCRIPTION
1.	1. Eggs (3) 1 portion = 20 grams protein and 270 calories. 2. Vegetable serving = 75 calories and 6 grams fiber. 3. Fruit serving = 75 calories and 3 grams fiber.
2.	1. OBNS Protein Supplement 1 portion = 15 grams protein, 160 calories, and 3 grams fiber. 2. Fruit serving = 75 calories and 3 grams fiber. 3. Sliced meat 1 portion = 20 grams protein and 100 calories.
3.	1. Sliced meat 2 portions =40g protein and 200 calories. 2. Vegetables 2 servings = 150 calories and 6 grams fiber. 3. Fruit serving = 75 calories and 3 grams fiber.
4.	1. OBNS Protein Supplement 1 portion =20 grams protein, 110 calories and 3 grams fiber. 2. Fruit serving = 75 calories and 3 grams fiber.
5.	1. Protein Pasta with lean meat sauce 2 portions = 40 grams protein and 200 calories. 2. Vegetables 2 servings = 150 calories and 6 grams fiber. 3. Fruit 1 servings = 75 calories, 6 grams of fiber.
6.	1. Sliced meat 2 portion =40 grams protein and 200 calories. 2. Fruit serving = 75 calories and 3 grams fiber **Totals: Protein 190 grams in 10 portions, Calories 2065, fiber 45 grams, Yellow carbs 0 grams**

DAY 6

MEAL	DESCRIPTION
1.	1. OBNS Protein Supplement 1 portion = 20 grams protein, 110 calories, and 5 grams fiber 2. Vegetable serving = 75 calories and 3 grams fiber. 3. Fruit 2 servings = 150 calories and 6 grams fiber.
2.	1. OBNS Protein Supplement 1 portion = 15 grams protein, 160 calories, and 3 grams fiber. 2. Fruit serving = 75 calories and 3 grams fiber. 3. Sliced meat 1 portion = 20 grams protein and 100 calories.
3.	1. Sliced meat 2 portions =40g protein and 200 calories. 2. Vegetables 2 servings = 150 calories and 6 grams fiber. 3. Fruit serving = 75 calories and 3 grams fiber.
4.	1. OBNS Protein Supplement 1 portion =20 grams protein, 110 calories and 3 grams fiber. 2. Fruit serving = 75 calories and 3 grams fiber.
5.	1. Grilled Salmon 2 portions = 40 grams protein and 200 calories. 2. Vegetables 2 servings = 150 calories and 6 grams fiber. 3. Fruit 1 servings = 75 calories, 3 grams of fiber.
6.	1. Sliced meat 2 portion =40 grams protein and 200 calories. 2. Fruit 2 servings = 150 calories and 6 grams fiber **Totals: Protein 190 grams in 10 portions, Calories 2055, fiber 50 grams, Yellow carbs 0 grams**

OB NUTRITIONAL SYSTEMS SAMPLE MENUS
SECOND TRIMESTER: 35 y/o, 5'4", 150 pound Sedentary Woman
DAY 7

MEAL	DESCRIPTION
1.	1. OBNS Protein Supplement 1 portion = 20 grams protein, 120 calories, and 5 grams fiber 2. Vegetable serving = 75 calories and 3 grams fiber. 3. Fruit 1 servings = 75 calories and 6 grams fiber.
2.	1. OBNS Protein Supplement 1 portion = 15 grams protein, 160 calories, and 3 grams fiber. 2. Fruit serving = 75 calories and 3 grams fiber. 3. Sliced meat 1 portion = 20 grams protein and 100 calories.
3.	1. Sliced meat 2 portions =40g protein and 200 calories. 2. Vegetables 1 servings = 75 calories and 6 grams fiber. 3. Fruit serving = 75 calories and 3 grams fiber.
4.	1. OBNS Protein Supplement 1 portion =20 grams protein, 120 calories and 3 grams fiber. 2. Fruit serving = 75 calories and 3 grams fiber.
5.	1. Steak 2 portions = 40 grams protein and 400 calories. 2. Vegetables 2 servings = 150 calories and 6 grams fiber. 3. Fruit 1 servings = 75 calories, 3 grams of fiber.
6.	1. Sliced meat 2 portion =40 grams protein and 200 calories. 2. 1 Fruit serving = 75 calories and 3 grams fiber **Totals: Protein 190 grams in 10 portions, Calories 2050, fiber 47 grams, Yellow carbs 0 grams**

BLANK MENUS
SECOND TRIMESTER
DAY 1

MEAL	DESCRIPTION
1.	
2.	
3.	
4.	
5.	
6.	

BLANK MENUS
SECOND TRIMESTER
DAY 2

MEAL	DESCRIPTION
1.	
2.	
3.	
4.	
5.	
6.	

BLANK MENUS
SECOND TRIMESTER
DAY 3

MEAL	DESCRIPTION
1.	
2.	
3.	
4.	
5.	
6.	

BLANK MENUS
SECOND TRIMESTER
DAY 4

MEAL	DESCRIPTION
1.	
2.	
3.	
4.	
5.	
6.	

BLANK MENUS
SECOND TRIMESTER
DAY 5

MEAL	DESCRIPTION
1.	
2.	
3.	
4.	
5.	
6.	

BLANK MENUS
SECOND TRIMESTER
DAY 6

MEAL	DESCRIPTION
1.	
2.	
3.	
4.	
5.	
6.	

G. Douglas Wood, MD

BLANK MENUS
SECOND TRIMESTER
DAY 7

MEAL	DESCRIPTION
1.	
2.	
3.	
4.	
5.	
6.	

13 THIRD TRIMESTER MINI PLANNER

OB Nutritional Systems Mini-Planner-Third Trimester Goals

During the third trimester you undoubtedly notice the increase in physical demands on your body as a result of the pregnancy. However, you have been preparing for this increase demand during your entire pregnancy by eating healthy and building lean muscle. By now you are feeling baby movements on a regular basis. With each movement comes the reassurance of a healthy baby; a baby that your healthy nutritional lifestyle has helped grow in a healthy way. Now that you have been eating healthy for close to six months, you can't help but see and feel the difference good nutrition makes in your wellbeing. You have avoided gaining any unnecessary weight from fat, and you have continued to increase lean muscle. All of which has made you stronger and healthier. You should have growing confidence in yourself, your pregnancy and your upcoming delivery.

Again, if you are just now joining us there is still time to reap some benefits. However, I recommend starting with the first trimester program adjusted for the increased calories, 150 extra calories for second trimester and another additional 150 calories in the third trimester. Then, after an abbreviated course of four to six weeks move up to the second trimester program for the remainder of the pregnancy.

In the third trimester you will increase your protein intake to 1.5 grams of protein per pound of body weight per day. This means you will have an additional 2 or 3 servings of protein per day. Make your selections from the lean, Green protein list or from protein supplements. You will avoid the Yellow and Red proteins.

In the third trimester you will also increase the minimum number of calories by 300 calories per day. In other words, an additional 150 calories from your second trimester amount. This is roughly the equivalent of four servings of fresh fruit or 10 graham crackers per day over your first trimester amounts. This will be enough additional calories to meet the increased metabolic demands of the pregnancy and your growing baby during your last trimester.

The Green carbohydrates continue to be unlimited, so enjoy them. You will reduce your Yellow carbohydrate intake to 1/2 gram per pound of body weight during the second trimester. For most of you this decrease should not be a problem, since most of you at this point have naturally moved significantly away from the Yellow carbohydrates already.

During the third trimester you will increase the minimum fiber intake to 50 grams. Again, if you are including a daily bowl of Fiber One cereal in your meal plan, then you will find it easier to meet this goal. You may even want to add additional ½ serving of Fiber One to help assure yourself of meeting your goal, since fiber helps you burn fat.

Now, review the OB Nutritional Systems Quick Guide and Daily Requirement pages for the third trimester to determine the protein, portion, and fiber requirements, and the yellow carbohydrate limit for your third trimester. Review the OB Nutritional Systems Base Calories for the third trimester along with the Height and Age Factor Calculator chart to obtain the values to include in the OB Nutritional Systems Calorie Worksheet for the third trimester. Add those numbers together to get your third trimester Prenatal Caloric Need. Then, use all the information to complete the daily requirements in your OB Nutritional Systems Daily Tracker. Afterward, update your favorites on the OB Nutritional Systems Personal Favorites chart. Again, using the sample menus, use your favorites list and other food items from the table to create your menus. By now, you should be very comfortable with this process and making your menus should come easy.

OB NUTRITIONAL SYSTEMS NUTRITION PLANNER QUICK GUIDE

------ THIRD TRIMESTER ------

Nutrient	
Protein	1.5 gram per pound of body weight
	Green protein: Your protein choices should come from these foods.
	Yellow protein: Avoid.
	Red protein: Avoid.
Carbohydrates	.5 gram per pound of body weight. (Up to maximum of 400g yellow carbohydrates per day.)
	Green carbohydrates: Unlimited, does not count toward your total.
	Yellow carbohydrates: Caution with these, stick within the limits.
	Red carbohydrates: Avoid. Special occasions only and count toward limit.
Fiber	50 grams
Prenatal Caloric Need	Base Calories Third Trimester + Age Factor + Height Factor

G. Douglas Wood, MD

OB NUTRITIONAL SYSTEMS DAILY REQUIREMENTS
THIRD TRIMESTER
Enter information for your weight in the OB Nutritional Systems Daily Tracker Third Trimester

3 ounces of protein = 20 usable grams of protein = 1 serving

(roughyl the size of a deck of playing cards)

Weight	Protein Grams	Protein Portions	Yellow Carb Limit Grams	Fiber Grams
70	105	5	35	50
80	120	6	40	50
90	135	7	45	50
100	150	8	50	50
110	165	8	55	50
120	180	9	60	50
130	195	10	65	50
140	210	11	70	50
150	225	11	75	50
160	240	12	80	50
170	255	13	85	50
180	270	14	90	50
190	285	14	95	50
200	300	15	100	50
210	315	16	105	50
220	330	17	110	50
230	345	17	115	50
240	360	18	120	50
250	375	19	125	50
260	390	20	130	50
270	405	20	135	50
280	420	21	140	50
290	435	22	145	50
300	450	23	150	50
310	465	23	155	50
320	480	24	160	50
330	495	25	165	50
340	510	26	170	50
350	525	26	175	50
360	540	27	180	50

OB NUTRITIONAL SYSTEMS BASE CALORIES

THIRD TRIMESTER

Enter the base calories for your weight and activity level in the OB Nutritional Systems Calorie Worksheet Third Trimester.

Weight	Sedentary	Lightly Active	Moderately Active	Very Active	Extra Active
70	1086	1200	1315	1429	1544
80	1141	1263	1386	1508	1630
90	1195	1325	1456	1586	1717
100	1250	1388	1527	1665	1803
110	1304	1450	1597	1743	1890
120	1359	1513	1668	1822	1976
130	1414	1575	1738	1900	2063
140	1468	1638	1809	1979	2149
150	1523	1701	1879	2057	2236
160	1578	1763	1950	2136	2322
170	1632	1826	2021	2214	2409
180	1687	1888	2091	2293	2495
190	1741	1951	2162	2371	2582
200	1796	2014	2232	2450	2668
210	1851	2076	2303	2528	2755
220	1905	2139	2373	2607	2841
230	1960	2201	2444	2685	2928
240	2015	2264	2514	2764	3014
250	2069	2326	2585	2842	3101
260	2124	2389	2655	2921	3187
270	2178	2452	2726	2999	3274
280	2233	2514	2797	3078	3360
290	2288	2577	2867	3156	3447
300	2342	2639	2938	3235	3533
310	2397	2702	3008	3313	3620
320	2452	2765	3079	3392	3706
330	2506	2827	3149	3470	3792
340	2561	2890	3220	3549	3879
350	2615	2952	3290	3627	3965
360	2670	3015	3361	3706	4052

OB NUTRITIONAL SYSTEMS HEIGHT AND AGE FACTOR CALCULATOR

Enter the height and age factors for your height and age in the OB Nutritional Systems Calorie Worksheet Third Trimester

Height	Height Factor		Age	Age Factor
4'0"	0		50	0
4'1"	22		49	6
4'2"	44		48	12
4'3"	66		47	18
4'4"	88		46	24
4'5"	110		45	30
4'6"	132		44	36
4'7"	154		43	42
4'8"	176		42	48
4'9"	198		41	54
4'10"	220		40	60
4'11"	242		39	66
5'0"	264		38	72
5'1"	286		37	78
5'2"	308		36	84
5'3"	330		35	90
5'4"	352		34	96
5'5"	374		33	102
5'6"	396		32	108
5'7"	418		31	114
5'8"	440		30	120
5'9"	462		29	126
5'10"	484		28	132
5'11"	506		27	138
6'0"	528		26	144
6'1"	550		25	150
6'2"	572		24	156
6'3"	594		23	162
6'4"	616		22	168
6'5"	638		21	174
6'6"	660		20	180
6'7"	682		19	186
6'8"	704		18	192
6'9"	726		17	198
6'10"	748		16	204
6'11"	770		15	210
7'0"	792		14	216
7'1"	814		13	222
7'2"	836		12	228

OB NUTRITIONAL SYSTEMS CALORIE WORKSHEET

------ THIRD TRIMESTER ------

Enter the Base Calories for your weight and activity level from the OB Nutritional Systems Base Calories Third Trimester table.	Base Calories = _____
Enter Height Factor for your height from the OB Nutritional Systems Height and Age Calculator.	Height Factor = _____
Enter Age Factor for your age from the OB Nutritional Systems Height and Age Calculator.	Age Factor = _____
Calculate **Prenatal Caloric Need**: Start with **Base Calories** and add the **Height Factor** and then add the **Age** and then enter the total as the **Prenatal Caloric Need**.	**Prenatal Caloric Need** = _____ Enter this number in the calorie goal on the OB Nutritional Systems Daily Tracker-Third Trimester.

OB NUTRITIONAL SYSTEMS DAILY TRACKER
YOUR DAILY REQUIRMENTS
THIRD TRIMESTER

Protein goal in grams: _____

Protein goal in servings: _____

Prenatal Caloric Need:_____

Yellow Carbohydrate limit in grams:_____

Fiber goal in grams:_____

		Meals 1	2	3	4	5	6	Totals	Total fiber
	Protein								
Day 1	Calorie								
	Carbs								
	Protein								
Day 2	Calorie								
	Carbs								
	Protein								
Day 3	Calorie								
	Carbs								
	Protein								
Day 4	Calorie								
	Carbs								
	Protein								
Day 5	Calorie								
	Carbs								
	Protein								
Day 6	Calorie								
	Carbs								
	Protein								
Day 7	Calorie								
	Carbs								

OB NUTRITIONAL SYSTEMS PERSONAL FAVORITES
THIRD TRIMESTER

Green Protein	Calories	Grams Protein	Green Carbohydrates	Calories	Grams Fiber
1			1		
2			2		
3			3		
4			4		
5			5		
6			6		
7			7		
8			8		
9			9		
10			10		

Protein Supplement	Calories	Grams Protein	Yellow Carbohydrates	Calories	Grams Fiber	Grams Carbs
1			1			
2			2			
3			3			
4			4			
5			5			
6			6			
7			7			
8			8			
9			9			
10			10			

Select your 10 favorite Green Proteins, Protein Supplements, Green Carbohydrates, and Yellow Carbohydrates. You can plan most of your meals with these. Keep track of calories on all items. Keep track of grams of protein for Green Protein and Protein Supplements. Keep track of grams of carbs on the Yellow Carbohydrates. (Don't Exceed Limit)

OB NUTRITIONAL SYSTEMS SAMPLE MENUS
THIRD   TRIMESTER: 35 y/o, 5'4", 150 pound Sedentary Woman
DAY 1

MEAL	DESCRIPTION
1.	1. Eggs (3) 1 portion = 20 grams protein and 270 calories. 2. Fiber One cereal 1 cup = 120 calories and 28 grams fiber. 3. Sliced meat 2 portion = 40 grams protein and 100 calories.
2.	1. OBNS Protein Supplement 1 portion = 15 grams protein, 160 calories, and 3 grams fiber. 2. Fruit serving = 75 calories and 3 grams fiber. 3. Sliced meat 2 portion = 40 grams protein and 200 calories.
3.	1. Sliced meat 2 portions =40g protein and 200 calories. 2. Vegetables 2 servings = 150 calories and 12 grams fiber. 3. Fruit serving = 75 calories and 3 grams fiber.
4.	1. OBNS Protein Supplement 1 portion =20 grams protein, 110 calories and 3 grams fiber. 2. Fruit serving = 75 calories and 3 grams fiber.
5.	1. Grilled Salmon 2 portions = 40 grams protein and 200 calories. 2. Vegetables 2 servings = 150 calories and 6 grams fiber. 3. Fruit 1 servings = 75 calories, 3 grams of fiber.
6.	1. Sliced meat 2 portion =40 grams protein and 200 calories. 2. Fruit serving = 75 calories and 3 grams fiber **Totals: Protein 190 grams in 12 portions, Calories 2235, fiber 65 grams, Yellow carbs 0 grams**

DAY 2

MEAL	DESCRIPTION
1.	1. OBNS Protein Supplement 1 portion = 20 grams protein, 110 calories, and 5 grams fiber 2. Fiber One cereal 1 cup = 120 calories and 28 grams fiber. 3. Sliced meat 2 portion = 40 grams protein and 100 calories.
2.	1. OBNS Protein Supplement 1 portion = 15 grams protein, 160 calories, and 3 grams fiber. 2. Fruit 2 servings = 150 calories and 6 grams fiber. 3. Sliced meat 2 portion = 40 grams protein and 200 calories.
3.	1. Sliced meat 2 portions =40g protein and 200 calories. 2. Vegetables 2 servings = 150 calories and 6 grams fiber. 3. Fruit serving = 75 calories and 3 grams fiber.
4.	1. OBNS Protein Supplement 1 portion =20 grams protein, 110 calories and 3 grams fiber. 2. Fruit serving = 75 calories and 3 grams fiber.
5.	1. Grilled Chicken 2 portions = 40 grams protein and 200 calories. 2. Vegetables 2 servings = 150 calories and 6 grams fiber. 3. Fruit 2 servings = 150 calories, 6 grams of fiber.
6.	1. Sliced meat 2 portion =40 grams protein and 200 calories. 2. Fruit 1 serving = 75 calories and 3 grams fiber **Totals: Protein 190 grams in 12 portions, Calories 2235, fiber 72 grams, Yellow carbs 0 grams**

OB NUTRITIONAL SYSTEMS SAMPLE MENUS
THIRD TRIMESTER: 35 y/o, 5'4", 150 pound Sedentary Woman
DAY 3

MEAL	DESCRIPTION
1.	1. Eggs (3) 1 portion = 20 grams protein and 270 calories. 2. Fiber One cereal 1 cup = 120 calories and 28 grams fiber. 3. Sliced meat 2 portion = 40 grams protein and 100 calories.
2.	1. OBNS Protein Supplement 1 portion = 15 grams protein, 160 calories, and 3 grams fiber. 2. Fruit serving = 75 calories and 3 grams fiber. 3. Sliced meat 2 portion = 40 grams protein and 200 calories.
3.	1. Tuna 2 portions =40g protein and 200 calories. 2. Vegetables 2 servings = 150 calories and 6 grams fiber. 3. Fruit serving = 75 calories and 3 grams fiber.
4.	1. OBNS Protein Supplement 1 portion =20 grams protein, 110 calories and 3 grams fiber. 2. Fruit serving = 75 calories and 3 grams fiber.
5.	1. Lean burger patties 2 portions = 40 grams protein and 200 calories. 2. Vegetables 2 servings = 150 calories and 6 grams fiber. 3. Fruit 1 servings = 75 calories, 6 grams of fiber.
6.	1. Sliced meat 2 portion =40 grams protein and 200 calories. 2. Fruit serving = 75 calories and 3 grams fiber **Totals: Protein 190 grams in 12 portions, Calories 2235, fiber 64 grams, Yellow carbs 0 grams**

DAY 4

MEAL	DESCRIPTION
1.	1. Eggs (3) 1 portion = 20 grams protein and 270 calories. 2. Fiber One cereal 1 cup = 120 calories and 28 grams fiber. 3. Sliced meat 2 portion = 40 grams protein and 100 calories.
2.	1. OBNS Protein Supplement 1 portion = 15 grams protein, 160 calories, and 3 grams fiber. 2. Fruit serving = 75 calories and 3 grams fiber. 3. Sliced meat 2 portion = 40 grams protein and 200 calories.
3.	1. Sliced meat 2 portions =40g protein and 200 calories. 2. Vegetables 2 servings = 150 calories and 6 grams fiber. 3. Fruit serving = 75 calories and 3 grams fiber.
4.	1. OBNS Protein Supplement 1 portion =20 grams protein, 110 calories and 3 grams fiber. 2. Fruit serving = 75 calories and 3 grams fiber.
5.	1. Grilled Chicken 2 portions = 40 grams protein and 200 calories. 2. Vegetables 2 servings = 150 calories and 6 grams fiber. 3. Fruit 1 servings = 75 calories, 6 grams of fiber.
6.	1. Sliced meat 2 portion =40 grams protein and 200 calories. 2. Fruit serving = 75 calories and 3 grams fiber **Totals: Protein 190 grams in 12 portions, Calories 2235, fiber 64 grams, Yellow carbs 0 grams**

OB NUTRITIONAL SYSTEMS SAMPLE MENUS
THIRD   TRIMESTER: 35 y/o, 5'4", 150 pound Sedentary Woman
DAY 5

MEAL	DESCRIPTION
1.	1. Eggs (3) 1 portion = 20 grams protein and 270 calories. 2. Fiber One cereal 1 cup = 120 calories and 28 grams fiber. 3. Sliced meat 2 portion = 40 grams protein and 100 calories.
2.	1. OBNS Protein Supplement 1 portion = 15 grams protein, 160 calories, and 3 grams fiber. 2. Fruit serving = 75 calories and 3 grams fiber. 3. Sliced meat 2 portion = 40 grams protein and 200 calories.
3.	1. Sliced meat 2 portions =40g protein and 200 calories. 2. Vegetables 2 servings = 150 calories and 6 grams fiber. 3. Fruit serving = 75 calories and 3 grams fiber.
4.	1. OBNS Protein Supplement 1 portion =20 grams protein, 110 calories and 3 grams fiber. 2. Fruit serving = 75 calories and 3 grams fiber.
5.	1. Protein Pasta with lean meat sauce 2 portions = 40 grams protein and 200 calories. 2. Vegetables 2 servings = 150 calories and 6 grams fiber. 3. Fruit 1 servings = 75 calories, 6 grams of fiber.
6.	1. Sliced meat 2 portion =40 grams protein and 200 calories. 2. Fruit serving = 75 calories and 3 grams fiber **Totals: Protein 190 grams in 12 portions, Calories 2235, fiber 64 grams, Yellow carbs 0 grams**

DAY 6

MEAL	DESCRIPTION
1.	1. OBNS Protein Supplement 1 portion = 20 grams protein, 110 calories, and 5 grams fiber 2. Fiber One cereal 1 cup = 120 calories and 28 grams fiber. 3. Sliced meat 1 portion = 20 grams protein and 100 calories.
2.	1. OBNS Protein Supplement 1 portion = 15 grams protein, 160 calories, and 3 grams fiber. 2. Fruit 2 servings = 150 calories and 3 grams fiber. 3. Sliced meat 2 portion = 40 grams protein and 200 calories.
3.	1. Sliced meat 2 portions =40g protein and 200 calories. 2. Vegetables 2 servings = 150 calories and 6 grams fiber. 3. Fruit serving = 75 calories and 3 grams fiber.
4.	1. OBNS Protein Supplement 1 portion =20 grams protein, 110 calories and 3 grams fiber. 2. Fruit serving = 75 calories and 3 grams fiber.
5.	1. Grilled Salmon 2 portions = 40 grams protein and 200 calories. 2. Vegetables 2 servings = 150 calories and 6 grams fiber. 3. Fruit 1 servings = 75 calories, 3 grams of fiber.
6.	1. Sliced meat 2 portion =40 grams protein and 200 calories. 2. Fruit 2 servings = 150 calories and 6 grams fiber **Totals: Protein 190 grams in 12 portions, Calories 2225, fiber 69 grams, Yellow carbs 0 grams**

OB NUTRITIONAL SYSTEMS SAMPLE MENUS
THIRD   TRIMESTER: 35 y/o, 5'4", 150 pound Sedentary Woman
DAY 7

MEAL	DESCRIPTION
1.	1. OBNS Protein Supplement 1 portion = 20 grams protein, 120 calories, and 5 grams fiber 2. Fiber One cereal 1 cup = 120 calories and 28 grams fiber. 3. Sliced meat 2 portion = 40 grams protein and 100 calories.
2.	1. OBNS Protein Supplement 1 portion = 15 grams protein, 160 calories, and 3 grams fiber. 2. Fruit serving = 75 calories and 3 grams fiber. 3. Sliced meat 2 portion = 40 grams protein and 200 calories.
3.	1. Sliced meat 2 portions =40g protein and 200 calories. 2. Vegetables 1 servings = 75 calories and 6 grams fiber. 3. Fruit serving = 75 calories and 3 grams fiber.
4.	1. OBNS Protein Supplement 1 portion =20 grams protein, 120 calories and 3 grams fiber. 2. Fruit serving = 75 calories and 3 grams fiber.
5.	1. Steak 2 portions = 40 grams protein and 400 calories. 2. Vegetables 2 servings = 150 calories and 6 grams fiber. 3. Fruit 1 servings = 75 calories, 3 grams of fiber.
6.	1. Sliced meat 2 portion =40 grams protein and 200 calories. 2. 1 Fruit serving = 75 calories and 3 grams fiber **Totals: Protein 190 grams in 12 portions, Calories 2220, fiber 66 grams, Yellow carbs 0 grams**

BLANK MENUS
THIRD TRIMESTER
DAY 1

MEAL	DESCRIPTION
1.	
2.	
3.	
4.	
5.	
6.	

BLANK MENUS
THIRD TRIMESTER
DAY 2

MEAL	DESCRIPTION
1.	
2.	
3.	
4.	
5.	
6.	

G. Douglas Wood, MD

BLANK MENUS
THIRD TRIMESTER
DAY 3

MEAL	DESCRIPTION
1.	
2.	
3.	
4.	
5.	
6.	

BLANK MENUS
THIRD TRIMESTER
DAY 4

MEAL	DESCRIPTION
1.	
2.	
3.	
4.	
5.	
6.	

BLANK MENUS
THIRD TRIMESTER
DAY 5

MEAL	DESCRIPTION
1.	
2.	
3.	
4.	
5.	
6.	

BLANK MENUS
THIRD TRIMESTER
DAY 6

MEAL	DESCRIPTION
1.	
2.	
3.	
4.	
5.	
6.	

BLANK MENUS
THIRD TRIMESTER
DAY 7

MEAL	DESCRIPTION
1.	
2.	
3.	
4.	
5.	
6.	

14 POSTPARTUM AND RECOVERY MINI PLANNER

OB Nutritional Systems Mini-Planner-Postpartum and Recovery Goals

Congratulations on your delivery! Now, it is really time to cash in on all the eating healthy and building lean muscle. You have probably noticed the demands on you are still there. They are just no longer inside you. He or she is now outside demanding all your attention. You have a lot going on, making adjustments for the new addition to the family. You should be up to the task, especially since you almost have your body back. In fact, if you were in fairly good shape to begin with and have been following the OB Nutritional Systems program during your entire pregnancy, then you won't have much to do, if any. Even if you weren't in the best shape to begin with, you are most likely in much better shape now having been eating healthy for the better part of nine months.

Those moms who are breast feeding will really turn up the fat burning now. You have been conditioning your body and making lean muscle for over the past nine months. Combine a lean conditioned body, with breast feeding, and you will quickly shed any remaining excess weight.

The next six weeks will cover the postpartum and recovery period. In the postpartum and recovery period you will no longer need the extra 300 calories per day. There are some conflicting recommendations that encourage an additional 500 calories for breast feeding. I don't think this is necessary with a healthy nutritional diet, since you are not calorie restricted. Regardless, the key factors with breast feeding are the nutritional quality of the food, adequate fluid intake, and emptying the breast of milk by feeding. These factors are much more important than the quantity of calories. Therefore, you will no longer need to track calories. You will notice that calories and the calorie worksheets have now been removed from your charts, tables, and menus. You will continue to consume 1.5 grams of protein per pound of body weight per day. You will also avoid the RED and Yellow proteins. The Green carbohydrates continue to be unlimited so enjoy them. You will continue to limit your Yellow carbohydrate intake to 1/2 gram per pound of body weight per day. You will also continue the minimum fiber intake to 50 grams.

Now, review the OB Nutritional Systems Quick Guide and Daily Requirement pages for the postpartum and recovery to determine how much protein and fiber you should eat and the limits on yellow carbohydrates. Then, use this information to complete the daily requirements in your OB Nutritional Systems Daily Tracker. Afterward, update your favorites on the OB Nutritional Systems Personal Favorites chart. Again, using the sample menus, use your favorites list and other food items from the table to create your menus. You know what to do.

OB NUTRITIONAL SYSTEMS NUTRITION PLANNER QUICK GUIDE

------ POSTPARTUM AND RECOVERY ------

Nutrient	
Protein	1.5 gram per pound of body weight Green protein: Your protein choices should come from these foods. Yellow protein: Avoid. Red protein: Avoid.
Carbohydrates	.5 gram per pound of body weight. (Up to maximum of 400g yellow carbohydrates per day.) Green carbohydrates: Unlimited, does not count toward your total. Yellow carbohydrates: Caution with these, stick within the limits. Red carbohydrates: Avoid. Special occasions only and count toward limit.
Fiber	50 grams

OB NUTRITIONAL SYSTEMS DAILY REQUIREMENTS
POSTPARTUM AND RECOVERY
Enter information for your weight in the OB Nutritional Systems Daily Tracker Postpartum and Recovery.

3 ounces of protein = 20 usable grams of protein = 1 serving

(roughyl the size of a deck of playing cards)

Weight	Protein Grams	Protein Portions	Yellow Carb Limit Grams	Fiber Grams
70	105	5	35	50
80	120	6	40	50
90	135	7	45	50
100	150	8	50	50
110	165	8	55	50
120	180	9	60	50
130	195	10	65	50
140	210	11	70	50
150	225	11	75	50
160	240	12	80	50
170	255	13	85	50
180	270	14	90	50
190	285	14	95	50
200	300	15	100	50
210	315	16	105	50
220	330	17	110	50
230	345	17	115	50
240	360	18	120	50
250	375	19	125	50
260	390	20	130	50
270	405	20	135	50
280	420	21	140	50
290	435	22	145	50
300	450	23	150	50
310	465	23	155	50
320	480	24	160	50
330	495	25	165	50
340	510	26	170	50
350	525	26	175	50
360	540	27	180	50

OB NUTRITIONAL SYSTEMS DAILY TRACKER
YOUR DAILY REQUIRMENTS
POSTPARTUM AND RECOVERY

Protein goal in grams: _____

Protein goal in servings: _____

Yellow Carbohydrate limit in grams: _____

Fiber goal in grams: _____

Meals

		1	2	3	4	5	6	Totals	Total fiber
	Protein								
Day 1	Calorie								
	Carbs								
	Protein								
Day 2	Calorie								
	Carbs								
	Protein								
Day 3	Calorie								
	Carbs								
	Protein								
Day 4	Calorie								
	Carbs								
	Protein								
Day 5	Calorie								
	Carbs								
	Protein								
Day 6	Calorie								
	Carbs								
	Protein								
Day 7	Calorie								
	Carbs								

G. Douglas Wood, MD

OB NUTRITIONAL SYSTEMS PERSONAL FAVORITES
POSTPARTUM AND RECOVERY

Green Protein	Calories	Grams Protein	Green Carbohydrates	Calories	Grams Fiber	
1			1			
2			2			
3			3			
4			4			
5			5			
6			6			
7			7			
8			8			
9			9			
10			10			

Protein Supplement	Calories	Grams Protein	Yellow Carbohydrates	Calories	Grams Fiber	Grams Carbs
1			1			
2			2			
3			3			
4			4			
5			5			
6			6			
7			7			
8			8			
9			9			
10			10			

Select your 10 favorite Green Proteins, Protein Supplements, Green Carbohydrates, and Yellow Carbohydrates. You can plan most of your meals with these. Keep track of calories on all items. Keep track of grams of protein for Green Protein and Protein Supplements. Keep track of grams of carbs on the Yellow Carbohydrates. (Don't Exceed Limit)

OB NUTRITIONAL SYSTEMS SAMPLE MENUS
POSTPARTUM AND RECOVERY: 150 POUND PERSON
DAY 1

MEAL	DESCRIPTION
1.	1. Eggs (3) 1 portion = 20 grams protein. 2. Fiber One cereal 1 cup = 28 grams fiber. 3. Sliced meat 2 portion = 40 grams protein
2.	1. OBNS Protein Supplement 1 portion = 15 grams protein and 3 grams fiber. 2. Fruit serving = 3 grams fiber. 3. Sliced meat 2 portion = 40 grams protein.
3.	1. Sliced meat 2 portions =40g protein. 2. Vegetables 2 servings = 12 grams fiber. 3. Fruit serving = 3 grams fiber.
4.	1. OBNS Protein Supplement 1 portion =20 grams protein, and 3 grams fiber. 2. Fruit serving = 3 grams fiber.
5.	1. Grilled Salmon 2 portions = 40 grams protein. 2. Vegetables 2 servings = 6 grams fiber. 3. Fruit 1 servings = 3 grams of fiber.
6.	1. Sliced meat 2 portion =40 grams protein. 2. Fruit serving = 3 grams fiber Totals: Protein 190 grams in 12 portions, fiber 65 grams, Yellow carbs 0 grams

DAY 2

MEAL	DESCRIPTION
1.	1. OBNS Protein Supplement 1 portion = 20 grams protein, 5 grams fiber 2. Fiber One cereal 1 cup = 28 grams fiber. 3. Sliced meat 2 portion = 40 grams protein.
2.	1. OBNS Protein Supplement 1 portion = 15 grams protein, and 3 grams fiber. 2. Fruit 2 servings = 6 grams fiber. 3. Sliced meat 2 portion = 40 grams protein.
3.	1. Sliced meat 2 portions =40g protein. 2. Vegetables 2 servings = 6 grams fiber. 3. Fruit serving = 3 grams fiber.
4.	1. OBNS Protein Supplement 1 portion =20 grams protein, and 3 grams fiber. 2. Fruit serving = 3 grams fiber.
5.	1. Grilled Chicken 2 portions = 40 grams protein. 2. Vegetables 2 servings = 6 grams fiber. 3. Fruit 2 servings = 6 grams of fiber.
6.	1. Sliced meat 2 portion =40 grams protein. 2. Fruit 1 serving = 3 grams fiber Totals: Protein 190 grams in 12 portions, fiber 72 grams, Yellow carbs 0 grams

OB NUTRITIONAL SYSTEMS SAMPLE MENUS
POSTPARTUM AND RECOVERY: 150 POUND PERSON
DAY 3

MEAL	DESCRIPTION
1.	1. Eggs (3) 1 portion = 20 grams protein. 2. Fiber One cereal 1 cup = 28 grams fiber. 3. Sliced meat 2 portion = 40 grams protein.
2.	1. OBNS Protein Supplement 1 portion = 15 grams protein, and 3 grams fiber. 2. Fruit serving = 3 grams fiber. 3. Sliced meat 2 portion = 40 grams protein.
3.	1. Tuna 2 portions = 40g protein. 2. Vegetables 2 servings = 6 grams fiber. 3. Fruit serving = 3 grams fiber.
4.	1. OBNS Protein Supplement 1 portion =20 grams protein, 3 grams fiber. 2. Fruit serving = 3 grams fiber.
5.	1. Lean burger patties 2 portions = 40 grams protein. 2. Vegetables 2 servings = 6 grams fiber. 3. Fruit 1 servings = 6 grams of fiber.
6.	1. Sliced meat 2 portion =40 grams protein. 2. Fruit serving = 3 grams fiber **Totals: Protein 190 grams in 12 portions, fiber 64 grams, Yellow carbs 0 grams**

DAY 4

MEAL	DESCRIPTION
1.	1. Eggs (3) 1 portion = 20 grams protein. 2. Fiber One cereal 1 cup = 28 grams fiber. 3. Sliced meat 2 portion = 40 grams protein.
2.	1. OBNS Protein Supplement 1 portion = 15 grams protein and 3 grams fiber. 2. Fruit serving = 3 grams fiber. 3. Sliced meat 2 portion = 40 grams protein.
3.	1. Sliced meat 2 portions =40g protein. 2. Vegetables 2 servings = 6 grams fiber. 3. Fruit serving = 3 grams fiber.
4.	1. OBNS Protein Supplement 1 portion =20 grams protein, and 3 grams fiber. 2. Fruit serving = 3 grams fiber.
5.	1. Grilled Chicken 2 portions = 40 grams protein. 2. Vegetables 2 servings = 6 grams fiber. 3. Fruit 1 servings = 6 grams of fiber.
6.	1. Sliced meat 2 portion =40 grams protein. 2. Fruit serving = 3 grams fiber **Totals: Protein 190 grams in 12 portions, fiber 64 grams, Yellow carbs 0 grams**

OB NUTRITIONAL SYSTEMS SAMPLE MENUS
POSTPARTUM AND RECOVERY: 150 POUND PERSON
DAY 5

MEAL	DESCRIPTION
1.	1. Eggs (3) 1 portion = 20 grams protein. 2. Fiber One cereal 1 cup = 28 grams fiber. 3. Sliced meat 2 portion = 40 grams protein.
2.	1. OBNS Protein Supplement 1 portion = 15 grams protein, and 3 grams fiber. 2. Fruit serving = 3 grams fiber. 3. Sliced meat 2 portion = 40 grams protein and 200 calories.
3.	1. Sliced meat 2 portions =40g protein. 2. Vegetables 2 servings = 6 grams fiber. 3. Fruit serving = 3 grams fiber.
4.	1. OBNS Protein Supplement 1 portion =20 grams protein, and 3 grams fiber. 2. Fruit serving = 3 grams fiber.
5.	1. Protein Pasta with lean meat sauce 2 portions = 40 grams protein. 2. Vegetables 2 servings = 6 grams fiber. 3. Fruit 1 servings = 6 grams of fiber.
6.	1. Sliced meat 2 portion =40 grams protein. 2. Fruit serving = 3 grams fiber **Totals: Protein 190 grams in 12 portions, fiber 64 grams, Yellow carbs 0 grams**

DAY 6

MEAL	DESCRIPTION
1.	1. OBNS Protein Supplement 1 portion = 20 grams protein and 5 grams fiber 2. Fiber One cereal 1 cup = 28 grams fiber. 3. Sliced meat 1 portion = 20 grams protein.
2.	1. OBNS Protein Supplement 1 portion = 15 grams protein, and 3 grams fiber. 2. Fruit 2 servings = 3 grams fiber. 3. Sliced meat 2 portion = 40 grams protein.
3.	1. Sliced meat 2 portions =40g protein. 2. Vegetables 2 servings = 6 grams fiber. 3. Fruit serving = 3 grams fiber.
4.	1. OBNS Protein Supplement 1 portion =20 grams protein and 3 grams fiber. 2. Fruit serving = 3 grams fiber.
5.	1. Grilled Salmon 2 portions = 40 grams protein. 2. Vegetables 2 servings = 6 grams fiber. 3. Fruit 1 servings = 3 grams of fiber.
6.	1. Sliced meat 2 portion =40 grams protein. 2. Fruit 2 servings = 6 grams fiber **Totals: Protein 190 grams in 12 portions, fiber 69 grams, Yellow carbs 0 grams**

OB NUTRITIONAL SYSTEMS SAMPLE MENUS
POSTPARTUM AND RECOVERY: 150 POUND PERSON
DAY 7

MEAL	DESCRIPTION
1.	1. OBNS Protein Supplement 1 portion = 20 grams protein, and 5 grams fiber 2. Fiber One cereal 1 cup = 28 grams fiber. 3. Sliced meat 2 portion = 40 grams protein.
2.	1. OBNS Protein Supplement 1 portion = 15 grams protein and 3 grams fiber. 2. Fruit serving = 3 grams fiber. 3. Sliced meat 2 portion = 40 grams protein.
3.	1. Sliced meat 2 portions =40g protein. 2. Vegetables 1 servings = 6 grams fiber. 3. Fruit serving = 3 grams fiber.
4.	1. OBNS Protein Supplement 1 portion =20 grams protein and 3 grams fiber. 2. Fruit serving = 3 grams fiber.
5.	1. Steak 2 portions = 40 grams protein. 2. Vegetables 2 servings = 6 grams fiber. 3. Fruit 1 servings = 3 grams of fiber.
6.	1. Sliced meat 2 portion =40 grams protein. 2. 1 Fruit serving = 3 grams fiber **Totals: Protein 190 grams in 12 portions, fiber 66 grams, Yellow carbs 0 grams**

BLANK MENUS
POSTPARTUM AND RECOVERY
DAY 1

MEAL	DESCRIPTION
1.	
2.	
3.	
4.	
5.	
6.	

BLANK MENUS
POSTPARTUM AND RECOVERY
DAY 2

MEAL	DESCRIPTION
1.	
2.	
3.	
4.	
5.	
6.	

BLANK MENUS
POSTPARTUM AND RECOVERY
DAY 3

MEAL	DESCRIPTION
1.	
2.	
3.	
4.	
5.	
6.	

BLANK MENUS
POSTPARTUM AND RECOVERY
DAY 4

MEAL	DESCRIPTION
1.	
2.	
3.	
4.	
5.	
6.	

BLANK MENUS
POSTPARTUM AND RECOVERY
DAY 5

MEAL	DESCRIPTION
1.	
2.	
3.	
4.	
5.	
6.	

BLANK MENUS
POSTPARTUM AND RECOVERY
DAY 6

MEAL	DESCRIPTION
1.	
2.	
3.	
4.	
5.	
6.	

BLANK MENUS
POSTPARTUM AND RECOVERY
DAY 7

MEAL	DESCRIPTION
1.	
2.	
3.	
4.	
5.	
6.	

15 MAINTENANCE MINI PLANNER

OB Nutritional Systems Mini-Planner- Maintenance Goals

YOU DID IT! You have made it through the pregnancy and postpartum period. You should feel proud of yourself, what an accomplishment. You have a healthy baby and a stronger, leaner, and healthier body. You will want to keep it that way and you can with the maintenance phase.

The maintenance phase is an ongoing process. During this time you will eat 1.25 grams of protein per pound of body weight per day. The strict avoidance of the Red and Yellow proteins is lifted slightly. Limit yourself to no more than 4 servings per week of Yellow proteins. You are no longer tracking calories. There are no calories on your charts, table and menus in this phase either.

The Green carbohydrates continue to be unlimited so enjoy them. You can now limit your Yellow carbohydrate intake to 1.5 grams per pound of body weight per day. Don't exceed your maximum. You will also continue taking fiber with a minimum fiber intake of 50 grams per day.

Now, review the OB Nutritional Systems Quick Guide and Daily Requirement pages for the maintenance phase and determine how much protein and fiber you should eat and the limits on yellow carbohydrates. Then, use this information to complete the daily requirements in your OB Nutritional Systems Daily Tracker. Afterward, update your favorites on the OB Nutritional Systems Personal Favorites chart. Again, using the sample menus, use your favorites list and other food items from the table to create your menus.

You might notice while looking at the menus that one day is different. One day is marked free. Everyone looks forward to the maintenance phase. That is because during this phase you get one free day a week. During this free day you can eat whatever you want. Yes, you heard right, whatever you want. You've earned it.

OB NUTRITIONAL SYSTEMS NUTRITION PLANNER QUICK GUIDE

------ MAINTENANCE ------

Nutrient	
Protein	1.25 gram per pound of body weight Green protein: Your protein choices should come from these foods. Yellow protein: Limit to 4 servings per week. Red protein: Avoid. Special occasions.
Carbohydrates	1.5 gram per pound of body weight. (Up to maximum of 300g yellow carbohydrates per day.) Green carbohydrates: Unlimited, does not count toward your total. Yellow carbohydrates: Caution with these, stick within the limits. Red carbohydrates: Avoid. Special occasions only and count toward limit.
Fiber	50 grams

G. Douglas Wood, MD

OB NUTRITIONAL SYSTEMS DAILY REQUIREMENTS
MAINTENANCE
Enter information for your weight in the OB Nutritional Systems

Daily Tracker Maintenance.

3 ounces of protein = 20 usable grams of protein = 1 serving

(roughyl the size of a deck of playing cards)

Weight	Protein Grams	Portions	Yellow Carb Limit Grams	Fiber Grams
70	105	5	35	50
80	120	6	40	50
90	135	7	45	50
100	150	8	50	50
110	165	8	55	50
120	180	9	60	50
130	195	10	65	50
140	210	11	70	50
150	225	11	75	50
160	240	12	80	50
170	255	13	85	50
180	270	14	90	50
190	285	14	95	50
200	300	15	100	50
210	315	16	105	50
220	330	17	110	50
230	345	17	115	50
240	360	18	120	50
250	375	19	125	50
260	390	20	130	50
270	405	20	135	50
280	420	21	140	50
290	435	22	145	50
300	450	23	150	50
310	465	23	155	50
320	480	24	160	50
330	495	25	165	50
340	510	26	170	50
350	525	26	175	50
360	540	27	180	50

OB NUTRITIONAL SYSTEMS DAILY TRACKER
YOUR DAILY REQUIRMENTS
MAINTENANCE

Protein goal in grams: _____

Protein goal in servings: _____

Yellow Carbohydrate limit in grams: _____

Fiber goal in grams: _____

Meals

		1	2	3	4	5	6	Totals	Total fiber
Day 1	Protein								
	Calorie								
	Carbs								
Day 2	Protein								
	Calorie								
	Carbs								
Day 3	Protein								
	Calorie								
	Carbs								
Day 4	Protein								
	Calorie								
	Carbs								
Day 5	Protein								
	Calorie								
	Carbs								
Day 6	Protein								
	Calorie								
	Carbs								
Day 7	Protein								
	Calorie								
	Carbs								

OB NUTRITIONAL SYSTEMS PERSONAL FAVORITES
MAINTENANCE

Green Protein	Calories	Grams Protein	Green Carbohydrates	Calories	Grams Fiber	
1			1			
2			2			
3			3			
4			4			
5			5			
6			6			
7			7			
8			8			
9			9			
10			10			

Protein Supplement	Calories	Grams Protein	Yellow Carbohydrates	Calories	Grams Fiber	Grams Carbs
1			1			
2			2			
3			3			
4			4			
5			5			
6			6			
7			7			
8			8			
9			9			
10			10			

Select your 10 favorite Green Proteins, Protein Supplements, Green Carbohydrates, and Yellow Carbohydrates. You can plan most of your meals with these. Keep track of calories on all items. Keep track of grams of protein for Green Protein and Protein Supplements. Keep track of grams of carbs on the Yellow Carbohydrates. (Don't Exceed Limit)

OB NUTRITIONAL SYSTEMS SAMPLE MENUS
MAINTENANCE: 150 POUND PERSON
DAY 1

MEAL	DESCRIPTION
1.	1. Eggs (3) 1 portion = 20 grams protein. 2. Vegetable serving = 6 grams fiber. 3. Fruit serving = 4 grams fiber.
2.	1. OBNS Protein Supplement 1 portion = 15 grams protein, and 3 grams fiber. 2. Fruit serving = 3 grams fiber. 3. Sliced meat 1 portion = 20 grams protein.
3.	1. Sliced meat 2 portions =40g protein. 2. Vegetables 2 servings = 12 grams fiber. 3. Fruit serving = 3 grams fiber.
4.	1. OBNS Protein Supplement 1 portion =20 grams protein and 4 grams fiber. 2. Fruit serving = 3 grams fiber.
5.	1. Grilled Salmon 2 portions = 40 grams protein. 2. Vegetables 2 servings = 6 grams fiber. 3. Fruit 1 servings = 4 grams of fiber.
6.	1. Sliced meat 2 portion =40 grams protein. 2. Fruit serving = 4 grams fiber **Totals: Protein 190 grams in 10 portions, fiber 50 grams, Yellow carbs 0 grams**

DAY 2

MEAL	DESCRIPTION
1.	1. OBNS Protein Supplement 1 portion = 20 grams protein, 5 grams fiber 2. Vegetable serving = 3 grams fiber. 3. Fruit 2 servings = 6 grams fiber.
2.	1. OBNS Protein Supplement 1 portion = 15 grams protein, 3 grams fiber. 2. Fruit 1 servings = 6 grams fiber. 3. Sliced meat 1 portion = 20 grams protein and 100 calories.
3.	1. Sliced meat 2 portions =40g protein. 2. Vegetables 2 servings = 6 grams fiber. 3. Fruit serving = 3 grams fiber.
4.	1. OBNS Protein Supplement 1 portion =20 grams protein, and 3 grams fiber. 2. Fruit serving = 3 grams fiber.
5.	1. Grilled Chicken 2 portions = 40 grams protein. 2. Vegetables 2 servings = 6 grams fiber. 3. Fruit 2 servings = 6 grams of fiber.
6.	1. Sliced meat 2 portion =40 grams protein. 2. Fruit 1 serving = 3 grams fiber **Totals: Protein 190 grams in 10 portions, fiber 53 grams, Yellow carbs 0 grams**

OB NUTRITIONAL SYSTEMS SAMPLE MENUS
MAINTENANCE: 150 POUND PERSON
DAY 3

MEAL	DESCRIPTION
1.	1. Eggs (3) 1 portion = 20 grams protein. 2. Vegetable serving = 6 grams fiber. 3. Fruit serving = 4 grams fiber.
2.	1. OBNS Protein Supplement 1 portion = 15 grams protein and 4 grams fiber. 2. Fruit serving = 4 grams fiber. 3. Sliced meat 1 portion = 20 grams protein.
3.	1. Tuna 2 portions =40g protein. 2. Vegetables 2 servings = 6 grams fiber. 3. Fruit serving = 3 grams fiber.
4.	1. OBNS Protein Supplement 1 portion =20 grams protein and 3 grams fiber. 2. Fruit serving = 4 grams fiber.
5.	1. Lean burger patties 2 portions = 40 grams protein. 2. Vegetables 2 servings = 6 grams fiber. 3. Fruit 1 servings = 6 grams of fiber.
6.	1. Sliced meat 2 portion =40 grams protein. 2. Fruit serving = 4 grams fiber **Totals: Protein 190 grams in 10 portions, fiber 50 grams, Yellow carbs 0 grams**

DAY 4

MEAL	DESCRIPTION
1.	1. Eggs (3) 1 portion = 20 grams protein. 2. Vegetable serving = 6 grams fiber. 3. Fruit serving = 4 grams fiber.
2.	1. OBNS Protein Supplement 1 portion = 15 grams protein and 5 grams fiber. 2. Fruit serving = 4 grams fiber. 3. Sliced meat 1 portion = 20 grams protein.
3.	1. Sliced meat 2 portions =40g protein. 2. Vegetables 2 servings = 6 grams fiber. 3. Fruit serving = 4 grams fiber.
4.	1. OBNS Protein Supplement 1 portion =20 grams protein and 3 grams fiber. 2. Fruit serving = 3 grams fiber.
5.	1. Grilled Chicken 2 portions = 40 grams protein. 2. Vegetables 2 servings = 6 grams fiber. 3. Fruit 1 servings = 6 grams of fiber.
6.	1. Sliced meat 2 portion =40 grams protein. 2. Fruit serving = 3 grams fiber **Totals: Protein 190 grams in 10 portions, fiber 50 grams, Yellow carbs 0 grams**

OB NUTRITIONAL SYSTEMS SAMPLE MENUS
MAINTENANCE: 150 POUND PERSON
DAY 5

MEAL	DESCRIPTION
1.	1. Eggs (3) 1 portion = 20 grams protein. 2. Vegetable serving = 6 grams fiber. 3. Fruit serving = 4 grams fiber.
2.	1. OBNS Protein Supplement 1 portion = 15 grams protein and 5 grams fiber. 2. Fruit serving = 4 grams fiber. 3. Sliced meat 1 portion = 20 grams protein.
3.	1. Sliced meat 2 portions =40g protein. 2. Vegetables 2 servings = 6 grams fiber. 3. Fruit serving = 4 grams fiber.
4.	1. OBNS Protein Supplement 1 portion =20 grams protein and 3 grams fiber. 2. Fruit serving = 3 grams fiber.
5.	1. Protein Pasta with lean meat sauce 2 portions = 40 grams protein. 2. Vegetables 2 servings = 6 grams fiber. 3. Fruit 1 servings = 6 grams of fiber.
6.	1. Sliced meat 2 portion =40 grams protein. 2. Fruit serving = 3 grams fiber **Totals: Protein 190 grams in 10 portions, fiber 50 grams, Yellow carbs 0 grams**

DAY 6

MEAL	DESCRIPTION
1.	1. OBNS Protein Supplement 1 portion = 20 grams protein, and 5 grams fiber 2. Vegetable serving = 3 grams fiber. 3. Fruit 2 servings = 6 grams fiber.
2.	1. OBNS Protein Supplement 1 portion = 15 grams protein and 3 grams fiber. 2. Fruit serving = 3 grams fiber. 3. Sliced meat 1 portion = 20 grams protein.
3.	1. Sliced meat 2 portions =40g protein. 2. Vegetables 2 servings = 6 grams fiber. 3. Fruit serving = 3 grams fiber.
4.	1. OBNS Protein Supplement 1 portion =20 grams protein, and 3 grams fiber. 2. Fruit serving = 3 grams fiber.
5.	1. Grilled Salmon 2 portions = 40 grams protein. 2. Vegetables 2 servings = 6 grams fiber. 3. Fruit 1 servings = 3 grams of fiber.
6.	1. Sliced meat 2 portion =40 grams protein. 2. Fruit 2 servings = 6 grams fiber **Totals: Protein 190 grams in 10 portions, fiber 50 grams, Yellow carbs 0 grams**

OB NUTRITIONAL SYSTEMS SAMPLE MENUS
MAINTENANCE: 150 POUND PERSON
DAY 7

MEAL	DESCRIPTION
1.	
2.	
3.	FREE DAY
4.	
5.	
6.	

BLANK MENUS
MAINTENANCE
DAY 1

MEAL	DESCRIPTION
1.	
2.	
3.	
4.	
5.	
6.	

BLANK MENUS
MAINTENANCE
DAY 2

MEAL	DESCRIPTION
1.	
2.	
3.	
4.	
5.	
6.	

BLANK MENUS
MAINTENANCE
DAY 3

MEAL	DESCRIPTION
1.	
2.	
3.	
4.	
5.	
6.	

BLANK MENUS
MAINTENANCE
DAY 4

MEAL	DESCRIPTION
1.	
2.	
3.	
4.	
5.	
6.	

G. Douglas Wood, MD

144

BLANK MENUS
MAINTENANCE
DAY 5

MEAL	DESCRIPTION
1.	
2.	
3.	
4.	
5.	
6.	

BLANK MENUS
MAINTENANCE
DAY 6

MEAL	DESCRIPTION
1.	
2.	
3.	
4.	
5.	
6.	

BLANK MENUS
MAINTENANCE
DAY 7

MEAL	DESCRIPTION
1.	
2.	
3.	**FREE DAY**
4.	
5.	
6.	

16 OB NUTRITIONAL SYSTEMS FOOD CHARTS

Here in part two of the OB Nutritional Systems Meal Planner you will find a list of various foods from which you will select and use to help plan your menus for all four cycles. You should be able to easily keep to these foods. However, you can also use foods that are not on this list as long as you can identify and confirm that they fall within a Green or Yellow classification, and you are able to locate nutritional information about the food item. If you are unable to decide which category or class a food item should be placed in, feel free to check on our website at **OBNutritionalSystems.com** or contact me at the following email address, **obnutritionalsystems@yahoo.com**, and I will help you.

In this section, you will find lists that contain the Green, Yellow, and Red categories of both proteins and carbohydrates. The protein foods are broken into color categories along with their approximate calories for each 20 grams of protein. Within each color category the proteins are subdivided into various classes of proteins. Each containing a group of similar types of related proteins. This has been done to help you find food choices faster. You will also notice that some proteins are denoted to be Super Green foods. Remember, these are Green proteins with the lowest fat content. The carbohydrate foods are likewise broken into similar color categories along with their approximate calories and fiber content. Within each color category the carbohydrates are also subdivided into various classes of carbohydrates. Each containing a group of similar types of related carbohydrates. Again, this should help you find food items faster.

The list of Red carbohydrates has been summarized. It would be impossible to list all the Red carbohydrates because our food supply is over whelmed with them. Because you are avoiding Red Proteins and especially Red carbohydrates you won't need as much detail as the other sections. I included them mainly to make you aware of their carbohydrate and calorie content. If you need the exact nutritional information on any item simply check the package. The nutritional information should be readily apparent.

GREEN PROTEINS

3 ounces of protein = 20 usable grams of protein= 1 serving (Roughly the size of a deck of playing cards)

BEEF
Average 200 calories per serving
All meats USDA select or choice and trimmed of fat.

Cubed steak	Filet mignon	Flank steak
Ground round, lean	Ground sirloin, lean	Round steak
Roast Beef	Sirloin steak	Tenderloin
Veal roast	Veal chop, lean	

DAIRY
Average 100 calories per serving

Cheese (<3 grams of fat per slice)	Grated Parmesan (2 tablespoons per portion)
Nonfat or low-fat cottage cheese*	Greek Yogurt 17g protein per 3.5 ounces

FISH
Average 100 calories per serving

Bass*	Bluefish	Catfish
Cod*	Crab	Flounder*
Haddock*	Herring	Halibut*
Imitation shellfish	Lobster	Mackerel
Orange roughy*	Oysters	Perch*
Pike*	Pollock*	Scallops*
Snapper*	Salmon	Sardines
Shrimp*	Swordfish	Trout
Tuna*	Turbot*	Whitefish*

GAME
Average 125 calories per serving
Without skin and drained of fat.

Buffalo*	Duck	Goose
Ostrich	Pheasant	Rabbit
Venison*		

*Denotes Super Green foods.

GREEN PROTEINS

3 ounces of protein = 20 usable grams of protein= 1 portion (Roughly the size of a deck of playing cards)

LAMB
Average 190 calories per serving

Chop	Leg	Roast

PORK
Average 180 calories per serving

Canadian bacon
Pork tenderloin

Lean ham   Loin Chop
Sausage (<1 gram of fat per ounce)

POULTRY
Average 105 calories per serving
White meat without skin.

Chicken*
Eggs
Turkey*

Cornish hen*   Deli meats (chicken or turkey 95% fat free)
Ground Chicken* Ground turkey*
Turkey or chicken hot dogs or sausage (<3 grams of fat per ounce)

*Denotes Super Green foods.

YELLOW PROTEINS

3 ounces of protein = 20 usable grams of protein= 1 serving (Roughly the size of a deck of playing cards)

BEEF
Average 250 calories per serving

Corned Beef	Ground beef (chuck)	New York strip
Porterhouse steak	Prime beef	Short ribs
T-bone steak	Veal cutlet	

DAIRY
Average 200 calories per serving

Feta cheese	Mozzarella cheese	Ricotta cheese
Cheese (<5 grams of fat per ounce)		

FISH
Average 275 calories per serving

Fried fish of any kind.

LAMB
Average 225 calories per serving

Rib roast	Ground

PORK
Average 250 calories per serving

Boston Butt	Loin-Top	Pork Chop
Pork cutlet	Sausage (= or <5 gram of fat per ounce)	

POULTRY
Average 150 calories per serving

Chicken, dark meat	Turkey, dark meat

SOY
Average 200 calories per serving

Soy milk	Tempeh	Tofu

151

RED PROTEINS

3 ounces of protein = 20 usable grams of protein= 1 serving (Roughly the size of a deck of playing cards)

BEEF
Average 300 calories per serving

Brisket   Prime rib roast   Rib steak
Sandwich meats (bologna, pimiento loaf, salami with 8 grams or more of fat per ounce)
Full-fat hot dogs (6-8 grams of fat per ounce)

DAIRY
Average 250 calories per serving

All regular full-fat cheeses (American, cheddar, Monterey Jack, Swiss)

NUTS
Average 250 calories per serving

All nuts   Nut butters

PORK
Average 300 calories per serving

Bacon   Bratwurst   Ground pork
Knockwurst   Pork sausage (Italian, Polish)   Spareribs
Full-fat pork hot dogs (6-8 grams of fat per ounce)

POULTRY
Average 250 calories per serving

Fried chicken   Chicken nuggets   Chicken Parmesan

GREEN CARBOHYDRATES		
With fiber content	Calories	Fiber grams
GRAINS		
All bran cereal (1cup)	120	31
Fiber One cereal (1 cup)	120	28.5
FRUITS		
Apple	100	4
Apple sauce, unsweetened (1cup)	100	3
Apricots	85	2
Avocado	80	10
Banana	105	3
Blackberries (1cup)	75	8
Blueberries (1cup)	110	4
Boysenberries (1cup)	75	5
Cantaloupe (1/2 melon)	80	2
Cherries (10)	85	3
Fig	75	2
Mango (1/2 small)	80	2
Nectarine	70	2
Orange	75	4
Papaya (1 cup)	75	2.5
Peach	70	2
Pear	75	4
Persimmon	75	6
Pineapple (1 cup)	75	2
Plum	100	1
Pomegranate	70	1
Raspberries (1 cup)	65	8
Strawberries (1 cup)	75	4
Tamarind	75	5
Tangerine	85	2
Watermelon (1 slice)	50	1.5
VEGETABLES-1 cup raw or ½ cup cooked		
Artichoke hearts	60	6
Arugula	60	.5
Asparagus	60	1.5
Bamboo shoots	70	3
Bean sprouts	70	1
Beets	75	4

Bell peppers	45	2
Bok Choy	50	1
Broccoli	85	3
Brussels sprouts	60	3
Cabbage	70	2
Carrots	70	4
Cauliflower	55	2.5
Celery	30	2
Cucumber	50	1
Endive	50	1.5
Eggplant	60	2
Fennel bulb	50	3
Jerusalem artichokes	60	2
Jicama	50	6
Kale	60	1.5
Kohlrabi	40	5
Leeks	40	2
Mushrooms	40	1
Mustard greens	40	2
Okra	60	3
Onion	60	3
Parsnips	50	7
Peas in the pod	70	2
Radishes	60	2
Salad greens	30	1
Sauerkraut	50	3.5
Scallions	50	3
Snow peas	70	2
Spinach	80	1
String beans	30	4
Sugar snap peas	50	2
Summer squash	60	2
Tomato	40	2
Tomato sauce	100	3.5
Turnips	60	2.5
Water chestnuts	60	3
Watercress	50	.5
Zucchini	60	1.5

YELLOW CARBOHYDRATES			
BREADS AND CRACKERS	Calories	Fiber grams	Carb grams
Animal crackers (8)	75	.22	15
Bagel	245	2	38
Bread, white (1 slice)	185	.5	13
Bread, whole wheat (1 slice)	70	2	13
Bread, rye (1 slice)	65	2	15.5
Bread, Italian (4 inches long)	145	1	15
Bread crumbs (1 cup)	427	1	22
Bread sticks (4 by ½ inch)	196	.15	3.5
Bun, hamburger or hotdog	177	1	22
English muffin	120	1.5	26
Graham cracker	30	.19	5
Matzo	111	1.5	22
Melba toast (4 slices)	50	1.25	15
Oyster crackers (24 crackers)	100	1	17
Pita (6 inch)	100	1.5	33.5
Pizza crust (1/2 6 inch pie)	225	3	32
Rice cakes (4 inch across, 2 cakes)	75	0	20
Roll	100	1	14
Saltines (2 crackers)	25	.18	4
Tortilla, corn (6 inch)	40	1.5	12
Tortilla, wheat (6 inch)	130	1.5	27
Wasa crisp bread (3 crackers)	60	2	11
Wasa flatbread (3 crackers)	60	2	11
Whole-wheat crackers (2crackers)	20	.25	4
CEREALS-1 cup cooked or ready to eat			
Granola	598	6	80
Grape-Nuts	210	10	94
Grits	145	.5	31
Kashi	140	2	13
Muesli	60	6.5	56
Oatmeal	30	2.5	16
Puffed cereals	60	.25	13
Shredded wheat	170	5.5	40
Special K	120	1	22.5
Wheat germ	30	14.5	56
Wheatena	480	6.5	29.
Wheaties	135	2.1	24

GRAINS-1 cup cooked

Amaranth	180	30	129
Barley	40	6	44
Bulgur	28	8	34
Couscous	200	2	36.5
Kamut	210	1	23
Kasha (buckwheat)	142	4.5	33.5
Millet	25	2.5	39
Pasta (regular)	180	2.5	39
Pasta (artichoke)	210	1	41
Pasta (spinach)	185	3	37
Rice (white)	205	.5	44.5
Rice(brown)	216	3.5	45
Quinoa	30	10	117
Wild rice	166	3	35

STARCHY VEGETABLES

Acorn squash (1 cup)	115	9	29
Beans, lentil, Pinto, black (1 cup)	30	16	40
butternut squash (1 cup)	82	6	24
Corn on the cob (1ear)	60	4	30
Hummus (1cup)	100	15	36
Idaho potato	130	2.5	34
potato, mashed (1cup)	237	4	35
pumpkin (1cup)	125	3	12
sweet potato	60	3.5	28
Yukon gold potato	130	2.5	34
Yams	150	5.5	38

SNACK FOODS

Popcorn (3 cups)	330	4.25	22
Potato Chips (light, 15-20 chips)	130	0	17
Pretzels (3/4 ounce)	75	1	17

RED CARBOHYDRATES

BEVERAGES
Average 150 calories per serving

All non-diet soda
Malted milk
Presweetened tea and fruit drinks and coffee drinks

Beer
Milkshakes- 525 calories

Hot Chocolate
Mixed alcoholic beverages
Wine

CEREALS-PRESWEETENED
Average 150 calories per serving

ALL varieties

CONDIMENTS
Average 50 calories per serving

Catsup
Molasses

Honey

Maple syrup

DESSERTS
Average 150 to 500 calories per serving

All cake
Cookies
Fruit snacks
Ice cream (fat and non-fat)
Presweetened packaged puddings

All pies
Cupcakes
Fruit rolls
Marshmallows

All Candy
Frozen yogurt
Fruit ice
Sorbet

SNACK FOODS
Average 150 calories per serving

Breakfast bars
Toaster pastry

Chips

Granola bars

17 EXERCISE AND PREGNANCY

The Benefits

Exercise during pregnancy is important. Being active and exercising on most, if not all, days of the week provides numerous health benefits for your health and the health of your pregnancy. You should exercise at least 30 minutes a day. Almost all pregnant women at some point in their pregnancy, will experience backaches, swelling, occasional constipation, and bloating. Exercise helps decrease and reduce the occurrence of these annoying symptoms. Becoming active and increasing muscle activity helps regulate blood sugar by increasing the uptake of glucose by the muscle and other cells. This synergistic effect on the body's insulin may help prevent or treat gestational diabetes. Pregnancy can be very taxing on your energy level. Stimulating your body with exercise and conditioning acclimates it to the increased demands of your pregnancy. Therefore exercise helps increase your energy. Mood changes can be a frequent side effect of pregnancy and is usually a consequence of feeling tired and drained. The improvement in energy that comes with exercising most certainly helps improve your mood. Engaging in regular exercise helps build muscle and improve muscle tone. Having good muscle and good muscle tone is necessary to help support your body's frame and posture while your center of gravity continues to move forward. All the increased muscle tone, strength, and endurance achieved with regular exercise is great during the day. What about at night? Being active and exercising regularly also helps you sleep better. The regular activity and exercise that will help keep you fit during pregnancy will also help improve your ability to cope with labor. By preparing yourself with exercise during your pregnancy, you will establish an excellent platform from which to start your endeavors on getting back into shape after the baby is born. Exercise during your pregnancy will certainly hasten your postpartum recovery.

There are changes which occur during pregnancy that you need to be aware of, because they may affect your exercise routine. There are hormones that get produced during pregnancy, which cause the ligaments that support your joints to become relaxed. This relaxation in the joints makes the joints more mobile. The increased mobility in the joints makes them more susceptible to injury. As pregnancy progresses, there is increasing weight in front of your body. This increased weight shifts your center of gravity forward, therefore places stress on joints and muscles. The areas of the body that tend to feel this stress more often are the pelvis and lower back. This is why these areas are common focuses of pain. This constant shifting forward of your center of gravity during pregnancy makes you less stable. The decrease in stability makes you more likely to lose your balance and fall. This becomes more prevalent as you progress through each trimester, especially in later pregnancy.

Another change for you to be aware of, your uterus increases in size along with the pregnancy and sits directly in front of the vena cava. The vena cava is a large blood vessel that returns the blood from the lower part of the body back to the heart. After the first trimester, the uterus is of sufficient size that it can partially compress the vena cava when you lay flat on your back. This can result in decreased blood return and an unpleasant drop in your blood pressure. This results in decreased blood flow to the pregnancy and other parts of body. The most immediate and noticeable side effects are lightheadedness, dizziness, and nausea with possible vomiting. Rolling on to your left side and getting off the flat of your back will quickly reverse the problem and symptoms. The best action here is prevention, therefore do not lay flat on your back after the first trimester.

During pregnancy, there are exercises and activities that are safe for you to participate in. There are exercises and activities you should avoid while you are pregnant. Walking is a good exercise for everyone. Swimming is also good for your body because it works so many muscles. Swimming also has the added benefit of relieving pressure on your back and joints, therefore giving them a much-needed break. Cycling and aerobics are good ways to improve your endurance and increase your heart rate, but be careful to keep your balance to avoid falls. Remember you're not as graceful as you were before pregnancy, because of your changing center of gravity. If you were a conditioned runner or accomplished ballerina before you became pregnant, you often can keep performing these activities during your pregnancy. You may however, have to modify or reduce your routine.

Strength training is an excellent form of exercise that has many benefits for you and your pregnancy. Strength training works in conjunction with and complements the healthy nutritional lifestyle that you plan to achieve. They work together to not only make you strong and healthy, but make you feel and look strong and healthy. Strength training will also improve and make you better at all the other physical activities and sports that you participate in. With strength training you increase your lean muscle mass and increase your fat burning ability. When you build muscle and burn fat you look leaner and healthier. Building muscle also helps you to gain healthy pregnancy weight and avoid unhealthy weight gain during your pregnancy. That is why strength training is the key subject in this section.

Any activity with a high risk of falling should be avoided during pregnancy. Such activities include gymnastics, waterskiing, and horseback riding. Racquet sports like tennis and racquetball should also be avoided because of the changing balance and the increased risk of falling. Downhill snow skiing not only has the risk of injuries and falls, it has the added risk of altitude sickness. Altitude sickness is an illness caused by breathing air that contains less oxygen. Contact sports should also be avoided, since these sports can result in harm to you and your baby. These sports include, but are not limited to: basketball, softball, soccer, and hockey. Scuba diving also has to be included in the activities to avoid. Scuba diving can put your baby at the risk of decompression sickness. This is a serious illness that can result from changes in the pressure surrounding the body.

There are a few conditions that you should be aware of when exercising during your pregnancy. There are certain positions and activities, because of your body changes, that may be risky for you and your baby. When you exercise, you should avoid activities that may strain joints and cause injury. Common activities like jumping, jarring motions or quick changes in direction can lead to these injuries and should be avoided. With increased activity comes the risk of becoming overheated, particularly in warmer climates. But, you can become overheated in cool climates as well. When you become overheated, you may cause the loss of fluids and become dehydrated. This can cause problems for your pregnancy. When you exercise you should follow certain guidelines to ensure a safe and healthy exercise program. As mentioned earlier, after the first trimester of pregnancy, avoid doing any exercises on your back. If you are unconditioned or have not exercised in a while, then you need to start slowly. You should start off as little as five minutes of exercise a day and gradually increase until you can stay active for 30 minutes a day. You should avoid brisk exercise in hot, humid weather. During hot seasons or in hot climates, exercise early in the morning or late in the evening when it is cooler. You can also exercise in a climate controlled facility such as a gym or athletic facility. You should avoid exercising if you have a fever, since the fever will already cause you to have an increase in body temperature. You should wear comfortable clothing that will help you remain cool. Investing in a bra that fits well and provides lots of support will help protect your breasts and help eliminate breast discomfort.

Your body uses water for multiple things including keeping itself cool and to avoid overheating. Therefore, you should drink plenty of water to help your body along and prevent dehydration. When outside be sure to protect sun exposed areas with adequate and proper sunscreen. Sunburn is not only unhealthy for your skin, but is extremely unpleasant when you are pregnant.

You should stop exercising immediately if you notice any of these warning signs. Vaginal bleeding may be incidental, but could signal a problem with your placenta. Placental abruption can be a serious problem. In most instances the bleeding is incidental, but notify you doctor if you have any vaginal bleeding. It is better to be safe than sorry. If you are dizzy or feel faint lie down on your left side immediately. This will usually resolve the symptoms immediately unless you're dehydrated. Regardless, take a break, hydrate, and inform your doctor. Chest pain always warrants further investigation and should be taken seriously. It may very well just be reflux and heartburn, but let your doctor decide. Stop immediately, rest and call your doctor. Headaches are common and nonspecific complaints. The cause is frequently fatigue and dehydration. Uncorrected vision and eye strain are also common triggers. Headaches can also result from blood pressure problems. Preeclampsia is a unique problem to pregnancy and can present with headaches. If headaches occur, rest, hydrate and notify your doctor. Muscle weakness can occur as a result of simple muscle fatigue but can result from dehydration or electrolyte imbalance. Appropriate hydration should correct the problem, but if it continues or reoccurs you should notify your doctor. Calf pain or swelling may result from injury or could be the symptom of a more serious clotting problem. Deep vein thrombosis, or DVT, can present with these symptoms and can result from injury to these areas or from dehydration or other undiagnosed problems. Get this checked out by your doctor. Uterine contractions, other than the occasional Braxton Hicks contractions, should be taken seriously. Stop exercising, rest, hydrate and notify your doctor. Leakage of fluid while exercising usually results from loss of urine, but it could be a loss of amniotic fluid. It is important to know the source of the leakage, because rupture of membranes warrants evaluation and treatment. If you are not sure, notify your doctor, again it is better to be safe than sorry.

Near the end of your second trimester you should be familiar with fetal kick counts and performing them regularly. If your baby is not passing the kick count test or if you are not feeling your baby move like you normally do then stop immediately and notify your doctor. If you are not familiar with fetal kick counts, there is plenty of information available online and you can discuss them with your doctor at your next prenatal visit.

Exercising during pregnancy not only prepares and helps you during your pregnancy, it also leaves you better prepared to start your postpartum recovery. If you have already been exercising, then you can gradually continue to increase and challenge yourself or build back to your pre-pregnancy routine. If you have not exercised during pregnancy, then start off slow and gradually build up and seriously consider strength building.

18 OB NUTRITIONAL SYSTEMS WORKOUT

A Simple System to Follow

OB Nutritional Systems Workout is a simple system to follow. It will help you keep your routine structured and efficient. You will save time and get fit without spending countless hours in the gym or on the treadmill. There are eighteen basic weight training exercises divided into four different workout sessions. Each workout session is performed once a week and each session should take less than an hour to complete. The OB Nutritional Systems Workout is divided into 4 phases. A phase for each of the trimesters of pregnancy and a postpartum recovery phase. The last phase can be continued indefinitely for maintenance. The phases use the same exercises except for occasional variations to account for the growing pregnancy. Some exercises cannot be performed or have to be modified after the first trimester. There are also some slight variations in the repetitions, amount of weights, and rest intervals. A repetition is a complete lift and return of the weight or complete movement and return on activities without weights. A repetition also includes completing the opposite side as well when opposite sides are worked independently of each other. A set is a group of repetitions that are performed without a rest.

The OB Nutritional Systems Workout can be tailored to your schedule. You can work out one session a day on any days of the week for 4 days. You can do this in any combinations of days. You can do 4 days in a row. You can do one day, skip a day, do two days, skip a day and then do the last day. You can do two days in a row, skip two days, and then complete the next two days. The point here is you can do them in any combination of days as you want as long as you complete each session once per week. If you only want to go to the gym twice a week then you can do two sessions each of the two days and complete your work out for the week. However you want to schedule your workout is fine; just complete the four sessions each week. Because you are only working each muscle group out once per week, there is built in rest time for each muscle group.

In each session you will find a description of the exercise and some photographs to help illustrate the exercise being performed and allow you to become more familiar with the equipment. You can work out any day of the week and at any time of the day. However, it is important to work the sessions in order and perform the exercises in order. The first session works out the chest and biceps. The second session works out the back and triceps. The third session works out the lower body and legs. Finally, the fourth session is dedicated to the shoulders and the abdominal muscles. The order the exercises are in is important too. The larger groups of muscles are worked out first, followed by independent muscle groups to minimize early fatigue on the small muscle groups. This will give you a more efficient workout.

Nearly all of the exercises in the OB Nutritional Systems Workout are to be performed on exercise machines. These machines should easily be found in most major gyms or health clubs. There are some alternate exercises shown in some cases in the event a machine is not available. A few alternates are to replace some of the exercises that cannot be performed after the first trimester. In most instances, the alternates will require free weights or an exercise band to perform. I recommend using the exercise machines whenever possible, because the machines keep you in the correct positions. This makes it easier for pregnant women since the hormones during pregnancy cause the supporting ligaments to become relaxed and more mobile. This increased mobility of the joints makes you more susceptible to injury with free weights if you are not careful.

You will probably notice a difference before too long, especially in your strength and tone. Your muscles will start to feel tighter and more compact. As you continue to progress, you will see your muscles become more defined under the skin as their over-lying fat dissolves and burns off from the combination of maintaining a healthy nutritional lifestyle and increasing efficiency of your muscles. To be successful with the OB Nutritional Systems Workout, you have to do it and be consistent. You cannot just breeze through the workouts with no effort or inadequate intensity and expect to get results. Don't just go through the motions or you will waste your time. Like everything else, you get out what you put in.

You don't need to struggle or be in pain, but you should be putting in effort. In fact, if you ever feel sharp pain, then stop what you are doing immediately. You may be doing something wrong or trying to lift too much and may have injured yourself. You should lift enough weight that by the time you are finishing your last repetitions on each set you should feel like you are working hard to finish.

On your very first day of each session plan to spend a little extra time to learn about the machines you will be using, and where they are located. Knowing how to adjust the seats and the weights and how each of them work will help you save time on future sessions. You may consult a personal trainer to help you if you are new to strength training. This will help you become more comfortable faster. If a personal trainer is not an option, most gyms and athletic clubs have a trainer on the floor to help answer questions for those using the equipment. Most gyms offer a free orientation to the equipment when you join, so keep that in mind if you plan to join a gym.

In the following pages, the exercise program is laid out with specific instructions for each of the four cycles. There is also a how to section with accompanying photographs to make the exercises easier and to help make you more comfortable with the equipment. You will also find workout charts for each phase. These are similar to the charts you will find in most gyms to help members track their progress. It will also quickly remind you of settings and amount of weight used for each exercise. You can make copies so you will have more. You can also download additional copies from our website at **OBNutritionalSystems.com** if you prefer.

If you plan to work out at home and without the use of exercise machines, then you will need to purchase a few items. A yoga mat will make floor exercises more comfortable and provide you with better traction when doing some of your exercises. You will need a good quality exercise band to perform most of your strength exercises. These are inexpensive and can be found at most sporting goods stores. I would get the type of exercise band that secures itself with a closed door, they are much safer than the plain stretch bands. The plain stretch bands that have you step on and pull or other similar type activities can slip and spring back hitting you in the face or abdomen. You don't want to hurt yourself or your unborn baby. Don't skimp here. A bar accessory for your exercise band will allow you to perform wide grip rows. Take care of your feet, buy a good pair of comfortable gym shoes to work out in.

Last is a set of weights. I would get a pair of 2 ½ and 5 pound dumbbell weights and an 8 pound medicine ball to start. Alternatively, if you familiarize yourself with the exercises before you buy, you might be able to try various weights at the store to see where your range is before buying.

A note about abdominal, lower body and leg exercises. The abdominal exercises do not have any set number of reps. Simply do as many as you can in each set. In the case of planks, hold the position for as long as you can. Because several of the leg and lower body machines require you to lay on your back or stomach and are cramped at best, these have been omitted in favor of squats and lunges. Once you have delivered, I recommend that you add back the abdominal, leg curl, leg extension, calf raise and leg press exercise machines. I elected to omit these machines in the book to avoid confusion and accidental attempts at these machines by pregnant women. If you have been going to the gym during your pregnancy, you should be familiar and comfortable at the gym by delivery. You will, by that time, be able to locate and understand how to use those machines. If not, ask the resident gym trainer to show you. He will be glad to assist you. If you are working out at home then you will already be set. However, you can make a quick trip to the bookstore or jump online and find additional exercises to augment your work out at home if you prefer to take it up a notch.

General Instructions

The OB Nutritional Systems Workout is divided into 4 cycles. One for each trimester and one for the postpartum recovery period. Maintenance is accomplished by continuation of the fourth cycle. The general principals are the same for each cycle, but slight variations in each cycle allow for increasing progress and to account for your growing pregnancy along with its increased physical demands on your body. The exercise program works in conjunction with the meal plan to make sure that both aspects of the program support the goal of a healthier nutritional lifestyle and a body composition that will help you gain healthy pregnancy weight while avoiding unnecessary pregnancy weight.

OB Nutritional Systems operates on the principle of muscle exhaustion which leads to muscle growth. When you take the muscle to the limits of its capacity you force it to adapt and grow. Your objective is to take your muscle to the limits of its capacity and therefore stimulate a rapid growth in strength. As you progress through the cycles you will increase the repetitions and decrease the resting periods causing a more concentrated muscle exhaustion. This results in a subsequent build and repair process, which leads to muscle growth or hypertrophy. Increased growth means better fat burning ability and a healthier you.

Cycle 1: First Trimester.

In this phase you will establish basic exercise habits that will allow you to build the basic strength and muscle coordination that will help you feel better and obtain energy during the first part of your pregnancy. Simultaneously, you will be starting the ground work for a lifetime of better body composition. When you start this cycle, for each exercise, you need to determine your starting weight. To do this, start with a relatively light weight for you. If you can easily do 20 reps with a particular weight, then you need to move up in weight. Increase the weight by 25% until it gets more difficult. You can then add or subtract 5 or 10 % until you get to a weight that you can complete 6 reps with some effort. The weight should be heavy enough that you may barely finish the third set or you may be able to do only 4 or 5 reps. This will be your starting weight. You will stay with this weight until you can finish all 6 reps of each of your working set without struggling. Then, it is time to move up. A good rule of thumb is to increase your weight by 5-10%.

In the beginning you may see rapid progress and increases in strength. These rapid increases will soon level off and your progress, while just as real, will be less dramatic.

Cycle 2: Second Trimester.

This phase is dedicated to increasing muscle size and definition which will help you carry and cope with an ever growing uterus and baby. The increased muscle not only helps you offset the increase work your body has to do, but provides you with extra fat burning power to block unhealthy weight gain. This allows maximum room for healthy weight gain during your pregnancy. At the beginning of this cycle you will select your starting weight essentially the same way; but, this time you want to find the heaviest weight that you can lift 8 to 10 times with effort. As with cycle one, you may barely finish or fall short a few reps on the last set. You will probably be working with a lighter weight than you did in cycle 1, but don't worry; you are not going backwards. You are doing twice as many reps and a shorter rest period which fatigues the muscle faster and more completely. As your muscles fatigue in this cycle, you will feel like you are running out of gas towards the end of the reps. Once you are able to get through 10 reps without struggling it is time to increase your weight. Remember 5-10% increments is usually enough.

Cycle 3: Third Trimester.

This cycle concentrates the muscle you built to give you the needed strength and energy to complete your pregnancy and endure the process of delivery. At the beginning of this cycle you will select your starting weight essentially the same way, but this time you want to find the heaviest weight that you can lift 14 to 15 times with effort. As with cycle two, you may barely finish or fall short a few reps on the last set. You will probably be working with a lighter weight than you did in cycle 1 and 2. As before, you are fatiguing the muscles even faster and will feel like you are running out of gas. Once you are able to get through 15 reps without struggling, it is time to increase your weight. Remember 5-10% increments is usually enough.

Cycle 4: Postpartum and Recovery.

This cycle allows for the body's recovery from labor and delivery and continues, not only to recover, but build muscle and fat burning ability. These phases transition into a maintenance program to help continue and sustain healthy habits to maintain a healthy nutritional lifestyle. At the beginning of this cycle, you will select your starting weight essentially the same way as previous cycles. This time you want to find the heaviest weight that you can lift 6 times with effort. As with previous cycles, you may barely finish or fall short a few reps on the last set. This cycle is a little different. The number of reps are decreased the first 6 weeks to allow for a short break during postpartum and recovery. You may find that you continue with the weight from the last cycle or you may actually increase to a heavier weight since you are doing fewer reps. Increase the weight when you can do 6 reps without struggling.

After the first six weeks you will then transition into the maintenance phase by increasing reps to 12 and increasing the rest period to 2 minutes. Select starting weights and move up as you did with previous cycles.

CYCLE 1

First Trimester, 4 days a week

- 2 warm-up sets (light weight about 50-60% of your working weight).
- 3 working sets.
- 5 repetitions each set.
- Move up when you can finish the 5th repetition in the last set without struggling.
- 3 minute rest intervals.

CYCLE 2

Second Trimester, 4 days a week

- 2 warm-up sets (light weight about 50-60% of your working weight).
- 3 working sets.
- 10 repetitions each set.
- Move up when you can finish the 10th repetition in the last set without struggling.
- 2 minute rest intervals.

CYCLE 3

Third Trimester, 4 days a week

- 2 warm-up sets (light weight about 50-60% of your working weight).
- 3 working sets.
- 15 repetitions each set.
- Move up when you can finish the 15th repetition in the last set without struggling.
- 1 minute rest intervals.

CYCLE 4

6 weeks Postpartum and Recovery, 4 days a week

- 2 warm-up sets (light weight about 50-60% of your working weight).
- 3 working sets.
- 6 repetitions each set.
- Move up when you can finish the 6th repetition in the last set without struggling.
- 1 minute rest intervals.

CYCLE 4 Maintenance

Maintenance after recovery, ongoing, 4 days a week

- 2 warm-up sets (light weight about 50-60% of your working weight).
- 3 working sets.
- 12 repetitions each set.
- Move up when you can finish the 12th repetition in the last set without struggling.
- 2 minute rest intervals.

DAY 1

Chest and Biceps

1. Chest Press or alternate chest press (*alternate chest press not allowed after 1st trimester*)
2. Incline Press or alternate
3. Fly Maneuver or alternate
4. Dumbbell curl

DAY 2

Back and Triceps

1. Lat Pull Down or alternate
2. Seated Row or alternate
3. Seated Wide Grip Row or alternate
4. Triceps Push Down or alternate
5. Triceps Extension (*Triceps Extension not allowed after 1st trimester*) or alternate

DAY 3

Lower Body and Legs

1. Squats
2. Lunges
3. Leg Maneuvers

DAY 4

Shoulders and Abdominals

1. Shoulder Press or alternate
2. Seated Lateral Raise
3. Reverse Fly
4. Plank
5. Side Plank
6. Bird Dog

DAY 1 EXERCISE 1

CHEST PRESS

Muscle Group: Whole Chest

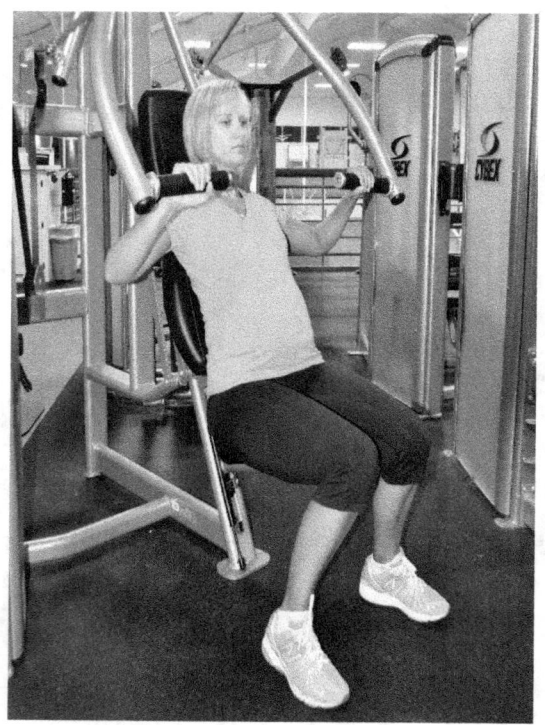 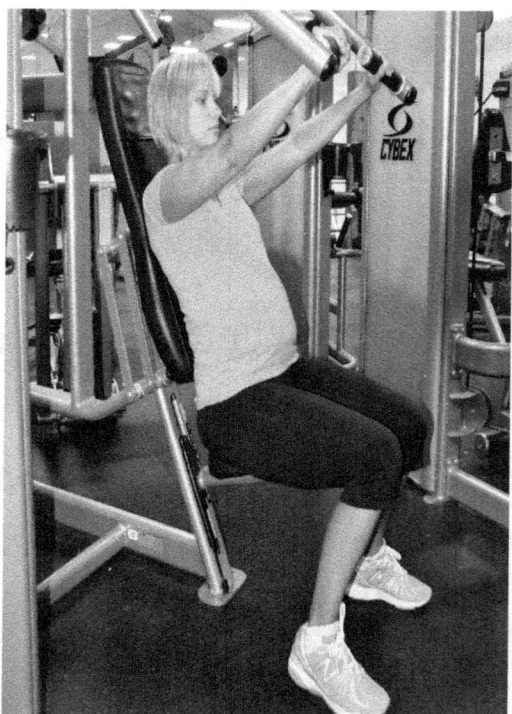

1. From the starting position, grip the handles with your hands about shoulder height and your elbows are raised to just below shoulder height.

2. Push the handles away until your arms are fully extended.

3. Return the handles to the starting position.

DAY 1 EXERCISE 1

ALTERNATE CHEST PRESS

Muscle Group: Whole Chest

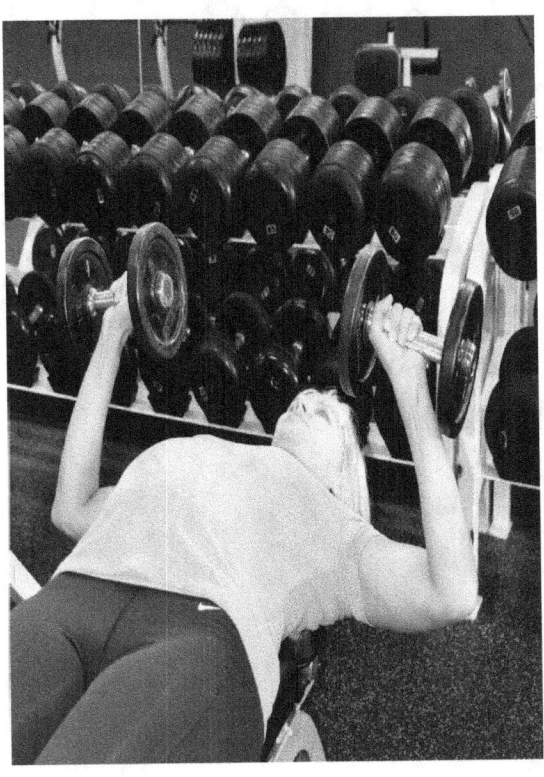 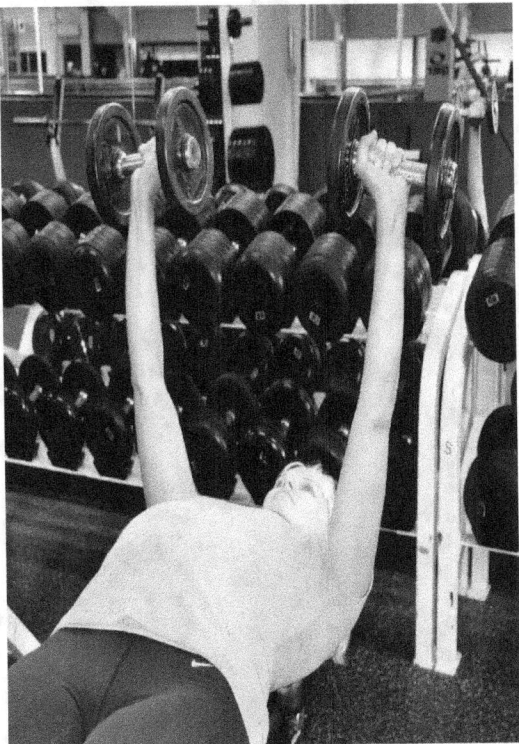

1. Lie flat on a bench (avoid after first trimester) with feet firmly on the ground.

2. From the starting position, hold the weights parallel to your shoulders and in line with your chest. Your elbows should make right angles.

3. Push the weights straight up until your arms are fully extended. The weights should be directly over each shoulder.

4. Slowly return the weights to the starting position.

DAY 1 EXERCISE 2

INCLINE PRESS

Muscle Group: Upper Chest

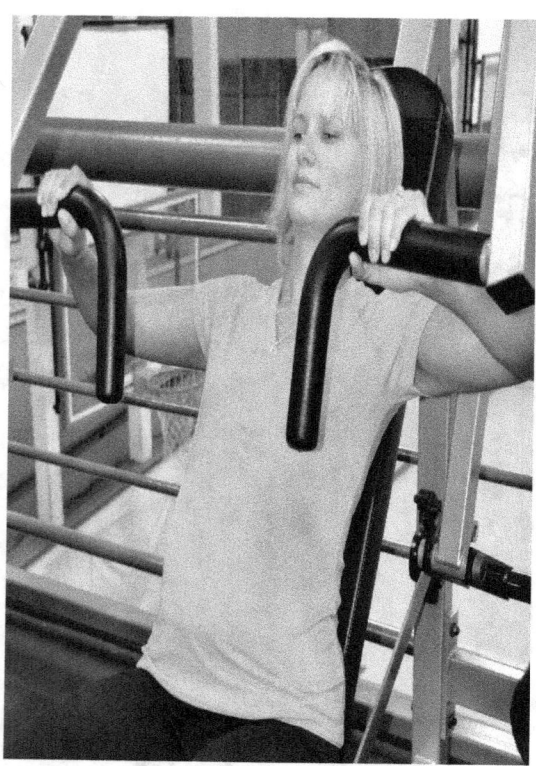 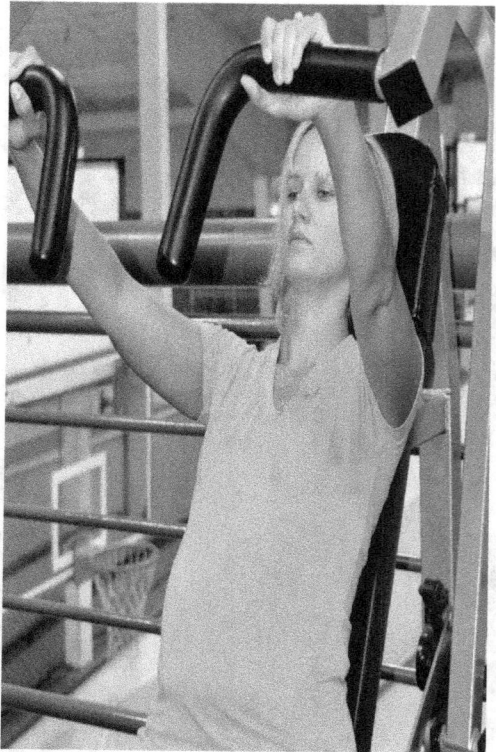

1. From the starting position, grip the handles with your hands about shoulder height and your elbows out to the sides.

2. Push the handles up until your arms are fully extended.

3. Return the handles to the starting position.

DAY 1 EXERCISE 2

ALTERNATE INCLINE PRESS

Muscle Group: Upper Chest

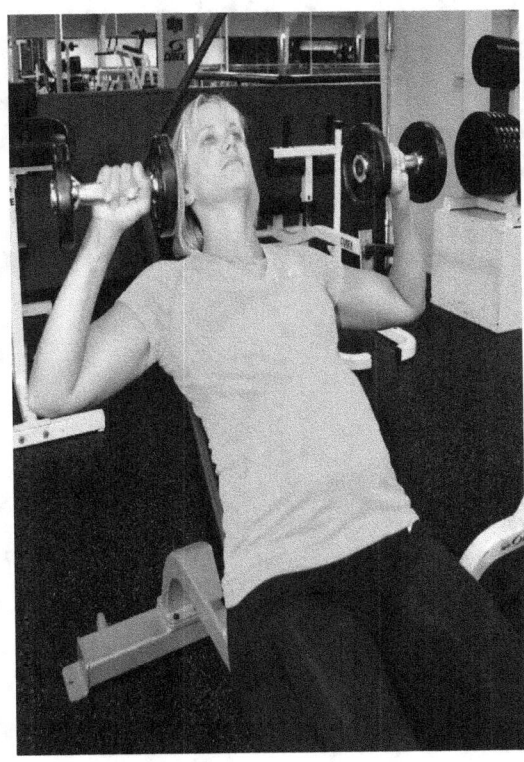 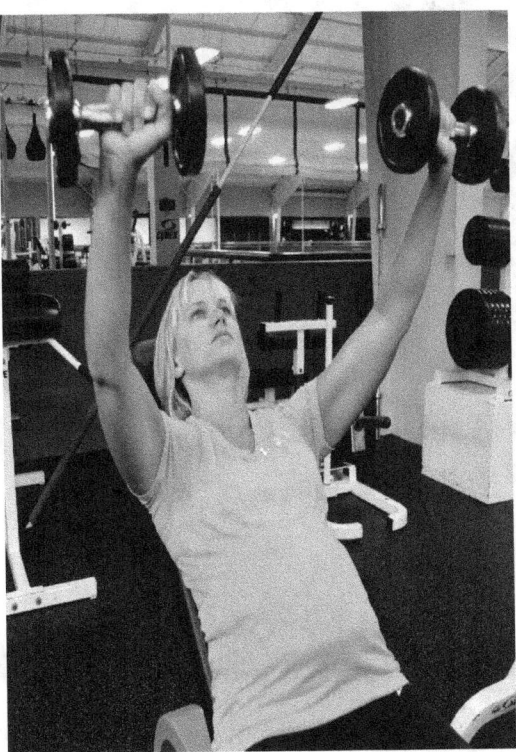

1. Lie on an incline bench at a 45 degree angle with your feet on the floor.

2. From the starting position, hold the weights with your elbows bent at a 90 degree angle. Your shoulders need to be in line with your collar bone.

3. Push the weights straight up over your chest until your arms are fully extended. The weights should be directly over each shoulder and not touching each other.

4. Slowly return the weights to the starting position.

DAY 1 EXERCISE 3

FLY MANEUVER

Muscle Group: Whole Chest

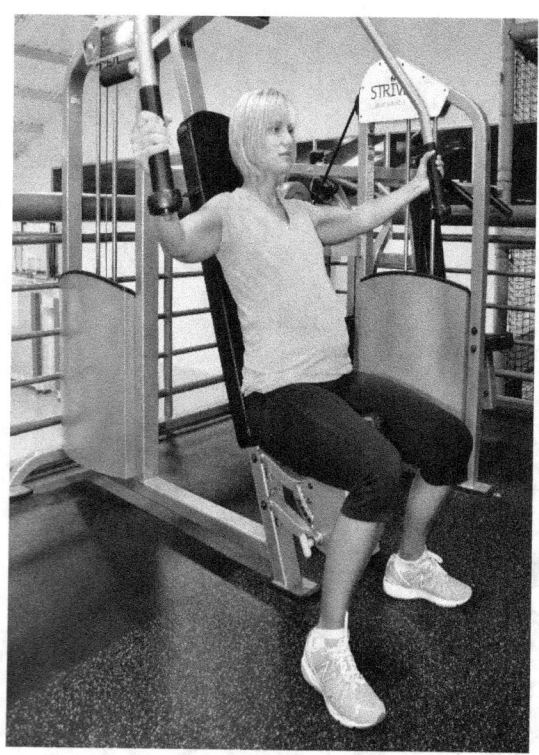 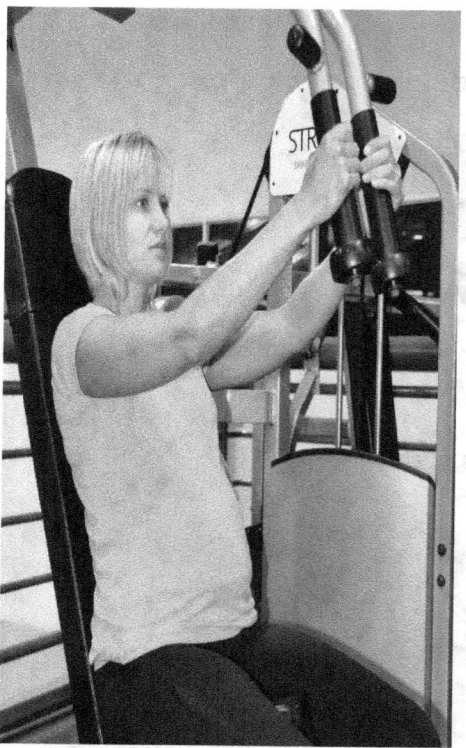

1. Adjust the seat so that your outstretched arms are at a 90 degree angle to your body when you grab the handles.

2. From the starting position, grip the handles with your hands and begin to move the handles forward.

3. Push the handles forward until your fists meet.

4. Slowly, return the handles to the starting position.

DAY 1 EXERCISE 3

ALTERNATE FLY MANEUVER

Muscle Group: Whole Chest

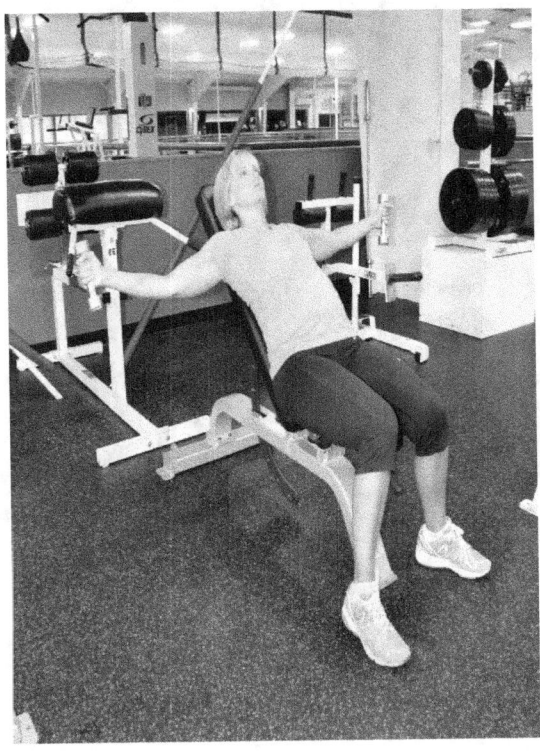 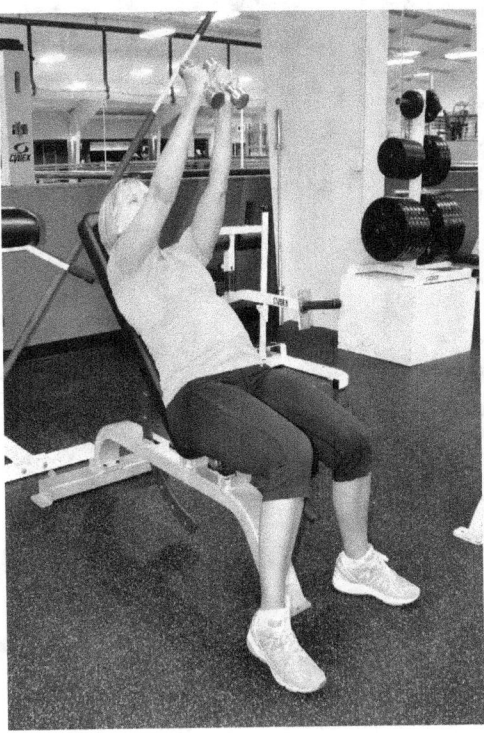

1. Lie on an incline bench at a 30 degree angle with your feet on the floor.

2. From the starting position, hold the weights parallel to your body and extend your arms. The elbows should be slightly bent.

3. Raise the weights over your chest while extending your elbows. Bring the weights together at the top.

4. Slowly return the weights to the starting position.

175

DAY 1 EXERCISE 4

DUMBELL CURL

Muscle Group: Biceps

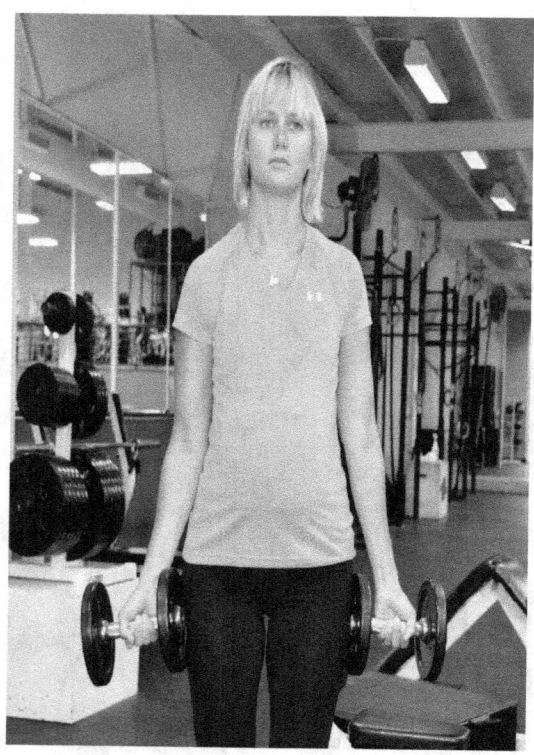 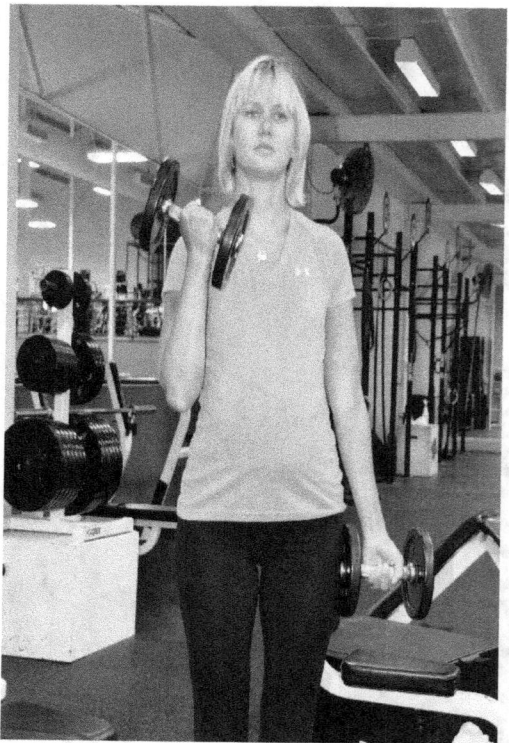

1. Stand straight with your feet placed shoulder width apart.

2. Grip one weight in each hand with your fists facing each other.

3. From the starting position, raise one arm at a time by bending at your elbow.

4. Bring the weight toward your shoulder.

5. Slowly, return the weights to the starting position.

6. Repeat the maneuver with the alternate arm to complete one repetition.

DAY 2 EXERCISE 1

LAT PULLDOWN

Muscle Group: Upper Back

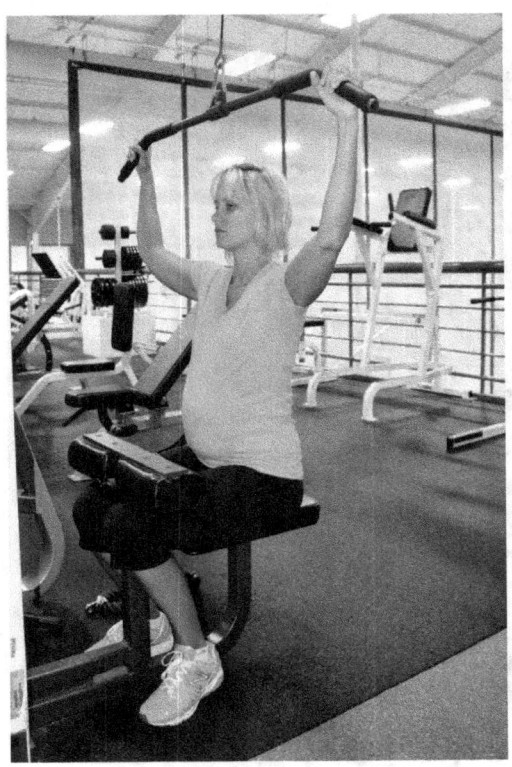 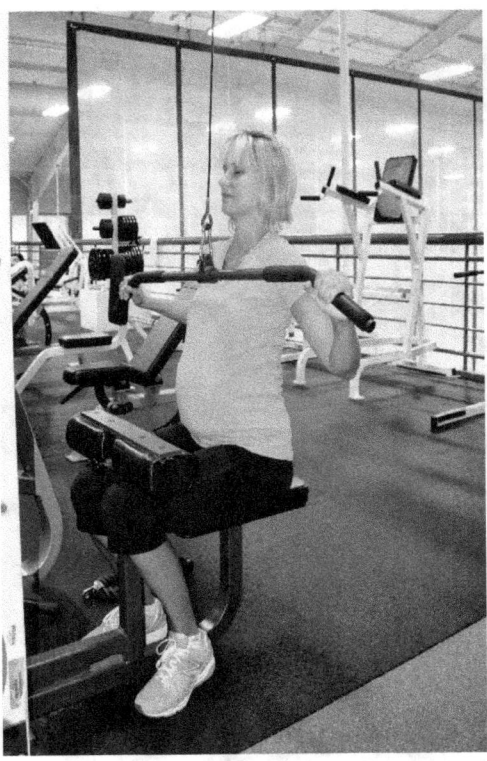

1. Sit on the bench with your legs firmly secured beneath the padding.

2. Reach up and grasp the bar. Hold it slightly wider than shoulder width.

3. From the starting position, your arms should be extended, pull the bar down to your collarbone. This should be slightly below your chin.

4. While you are pulling down the bar, concentrate on keeping your shoulders low and your chest forward.

5. Slowly return the bar to the starting position.

DAY 2 EXERCISE 1

ALTERNATE LAT PULLDOWN

Muscle Group: Upper Back

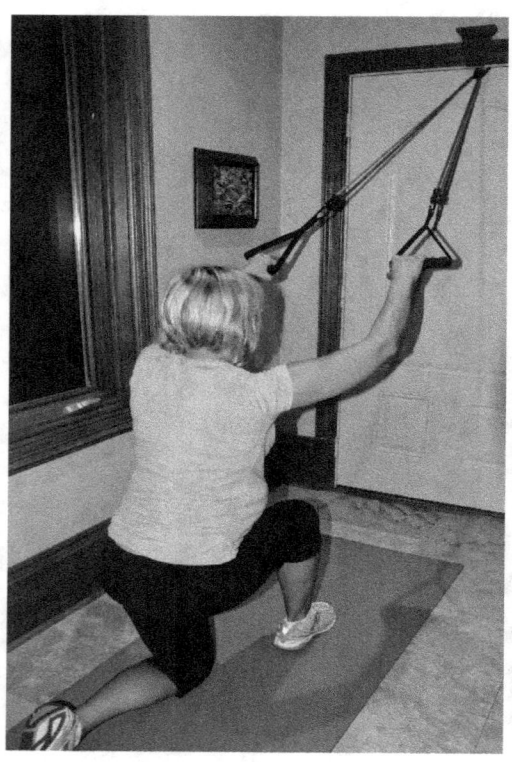 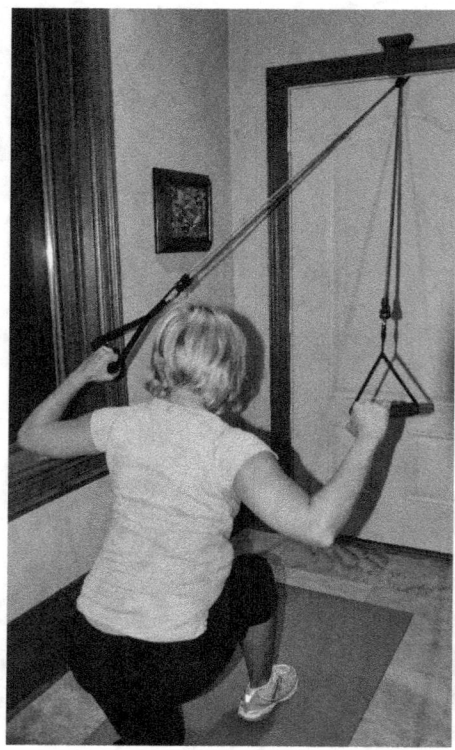

1.   Kneel down onto one knee and lean slightly forward.

2.   Grip one handle in each hand with your fists facing downward and arms extended.

3.   From the starting position, bring your arms parallel with your shoulders. While bringing your arms back, bend your elbows 90 degrees.

4.   Slowly, return to the starting position.

DAY 2 EXERCISE 2

SEATED ROW

Muscle Group: Lower Back

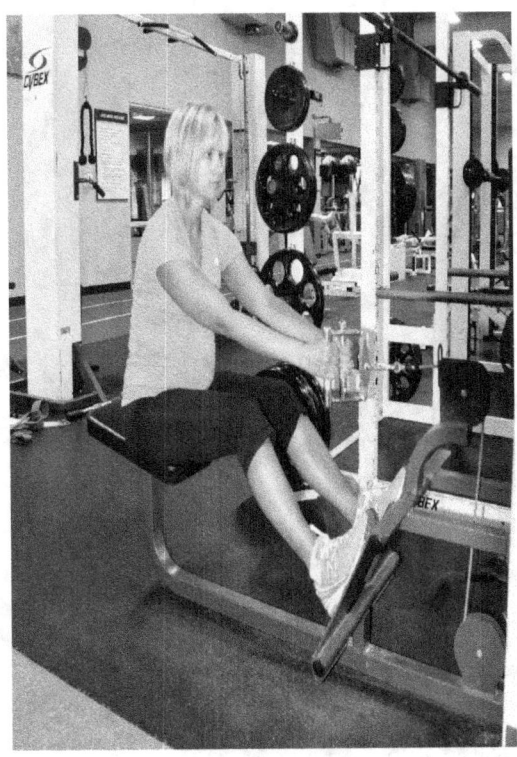 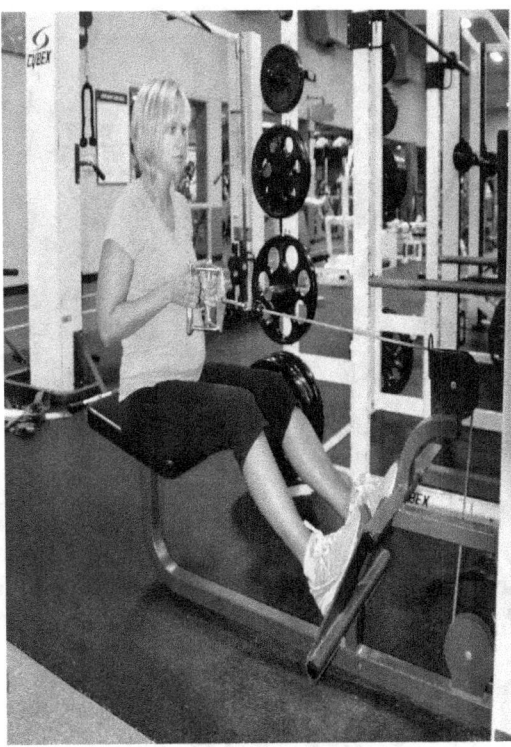

1. Start with your feet pressed against the footpad and your knees slightly bent.

2. Reach forward and grasp the handles. Bend at the waist and keep your back straight.

3. From the starting position, sit back to the upright position while your arms pull towards your lower abdomen.

4. Slowly return to the starting position.

G. Douglas Wood, MD

DAY 2 EXERCISE 2

ALTERNATE SEATED ROW

Muscle Group: Lower Back

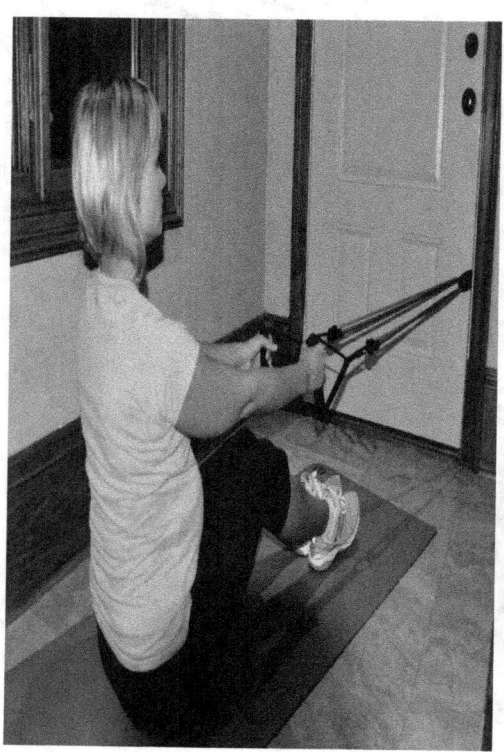 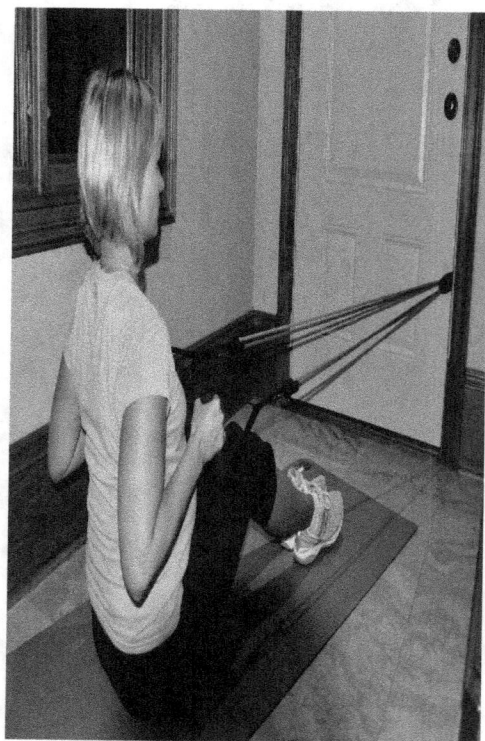

1. Start with your feet planted against the mat and your knees slightly bent.

2. Reach forward and grasp the handles. Bend at the waist and keep your back straight.

3. From the starting position, sit back to the upright position while your arms pull towards your lower abdomen.

4. Slowly return to the starting position.

180

DAY 2 EXERCISE 3

SEATED WIDE-GRIP ROW

Muscle Group: Whole Back

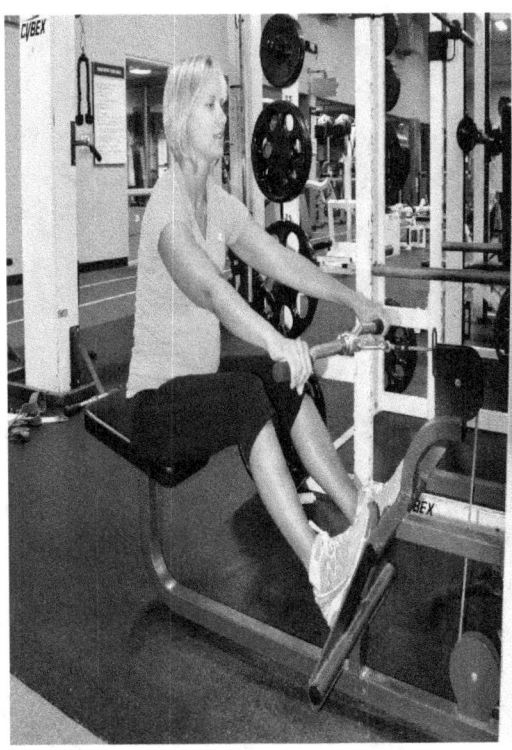 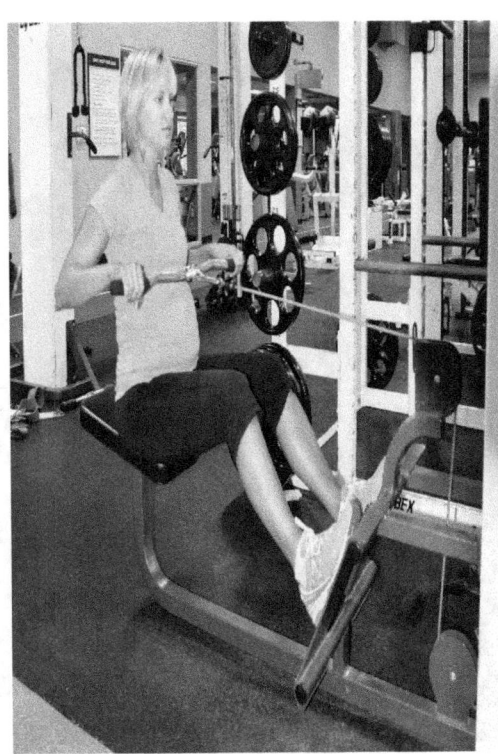

1. Start with your feet pressed against the footpad and your knees slightly bent.

2. Reach forward and grasp the horizontal bar. Hold the bar with your hands shoulder width apart. Bend at the waist and keep your back straight.

3. From the starting position, sit back to the upright position while your arms pull towards your lower abdomen. Your elbows should be flared outward at a right angle to your body.

4. Slowly return to the starting position.

DAY 2 EXERCISE 3

ALTERNATE SEATED WIDE-GRIP ROW

Muscle Group: Whole Back

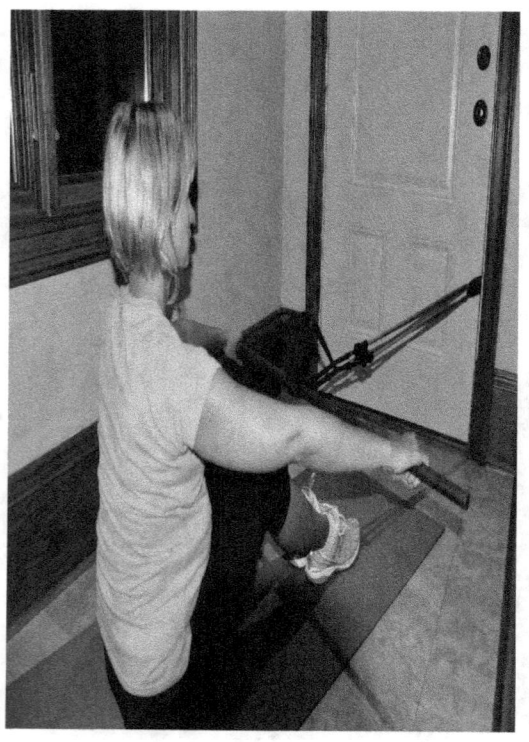 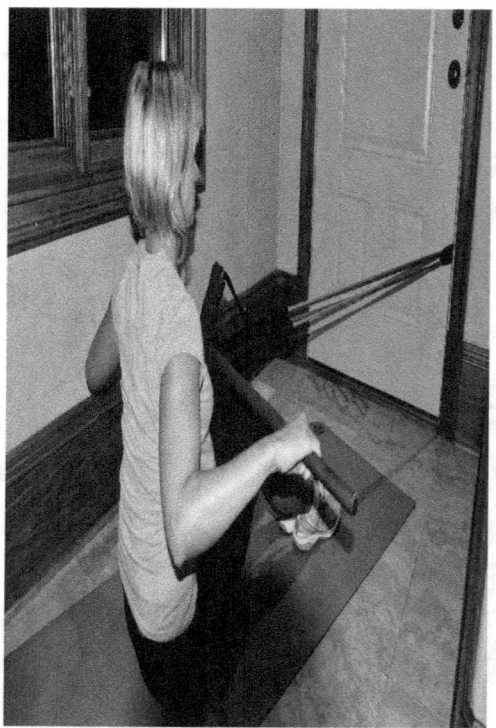

1. Start with your feet planted against the mat and your knees slightly bent.

2. Reach forward and grasp the horizontal bar. Hold the bar with your hands shoulder width apart. Bend at the waist and keep your back straight.

3. From the starting position, sit back to the upright position while your arms pull towards your lower abdomen. Your elbows should be flared outward at a right angle to your body.

4. Slowly return to the starting position.

DAY 2 EXERCISE 4

TRICEPS PUSHDOWN

Muscle Group: Triceps

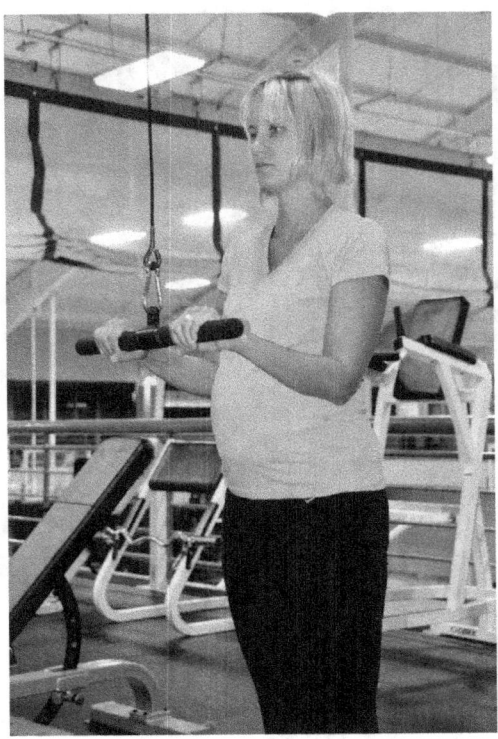 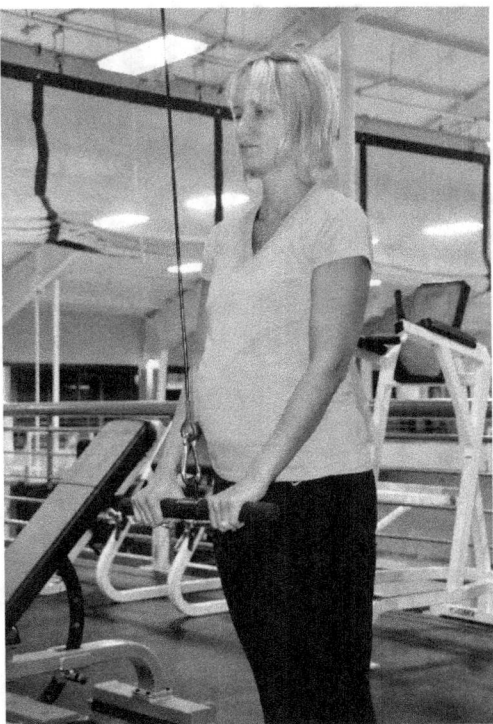

1. Start in the standing position. Grip the bar with your hands at hip width. Keep your elbows slightly bent.

2. From the starting position, push the bar straight down as far as you can.

3. Slowly return to the starting position.

DAY 2 EXERCISE 4

ALTERNATE TRICEPS PUSHDOWN

Muscle Group: Triceps

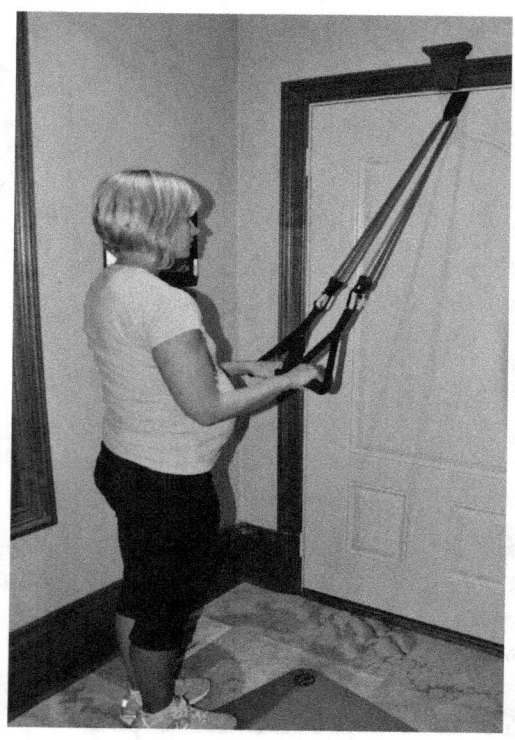 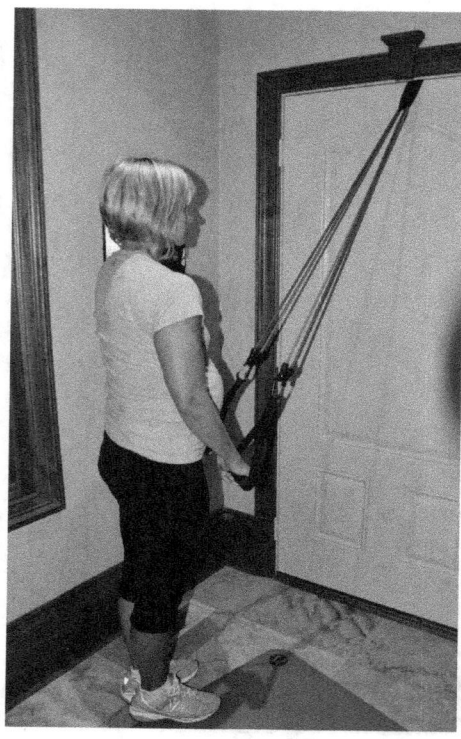

1. Start in the standing position. Grip the bar with your hands at hip width. Keep your elbows slightly bent.

2. From the starting position, push the bar straight down as far as you can.

3. Slowly return to the starting position.

DAY 2 EXERCISE 5

TRICEPS EXTENSION

Muscle Group: Triceps

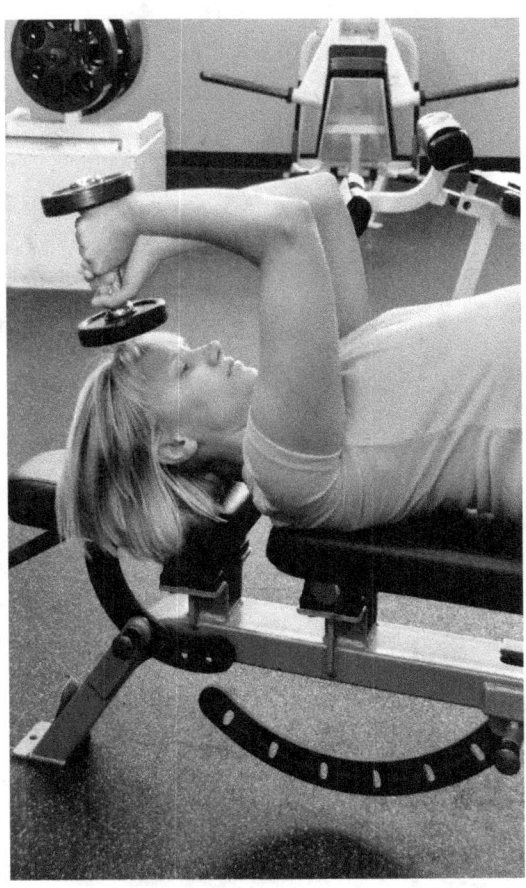 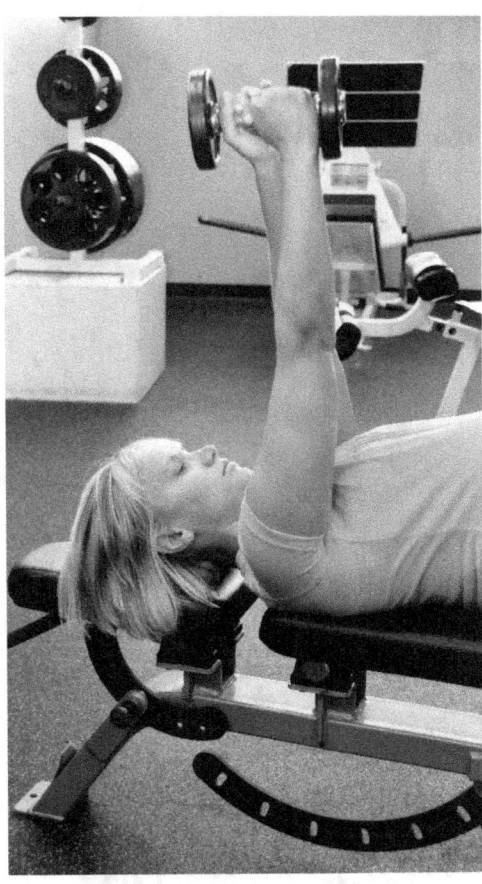

1. Lie flat on a bench (avoid after first trimester) with feet firmly on the ground.

2. With a weight in your hand, bend your arm into an L shape. The weight should be hovering over your forehead. Be careful not to hit your head.

3. Extend your arms completely straight up, bending only at the elbows.

4. Slowly return to the starting position.

DAY 2 EXERCISE 5

ALTERNATE TRICEPS EXTENSION

Muscle Group: Triceps

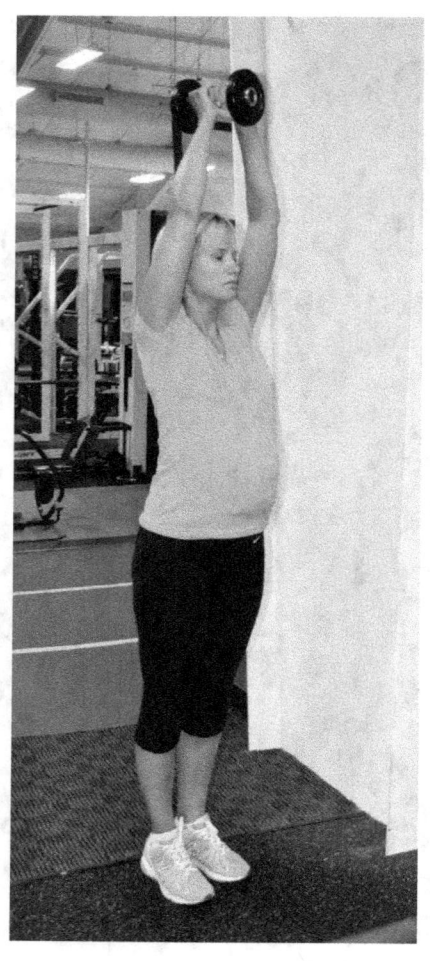 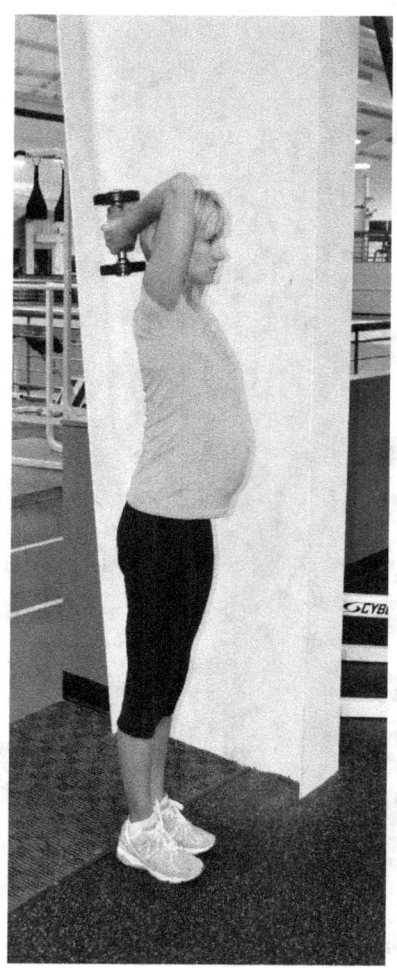

1. Start in a standing position.

2. With a weight in your hand, extend your arms straight over your head.

3. Bending only at the elbows, bend your arms back to a 90 degree angle.

4. Slowly return to the starting position.

DAY 3 EXERCISE 1

SQUATS

Muscle Group: Hamstrings, Calves, Quad, and Gluts

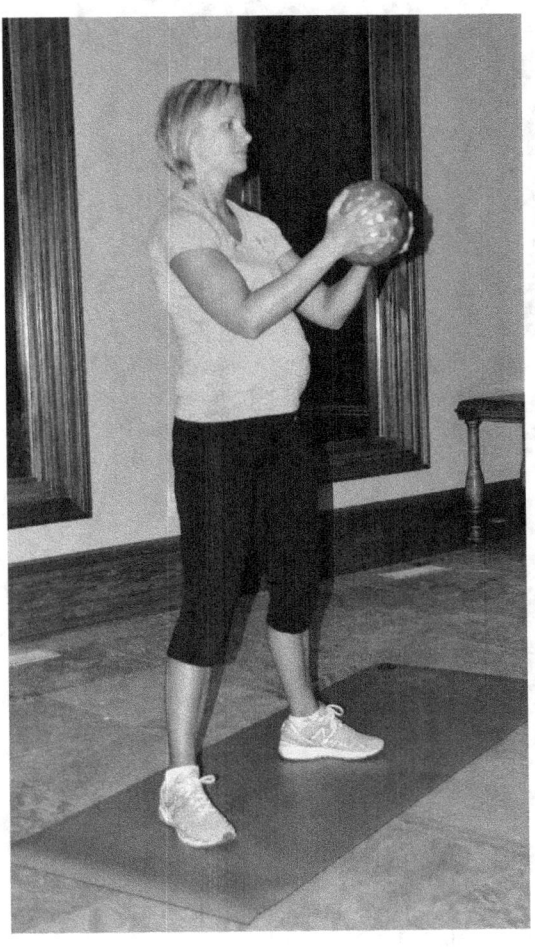 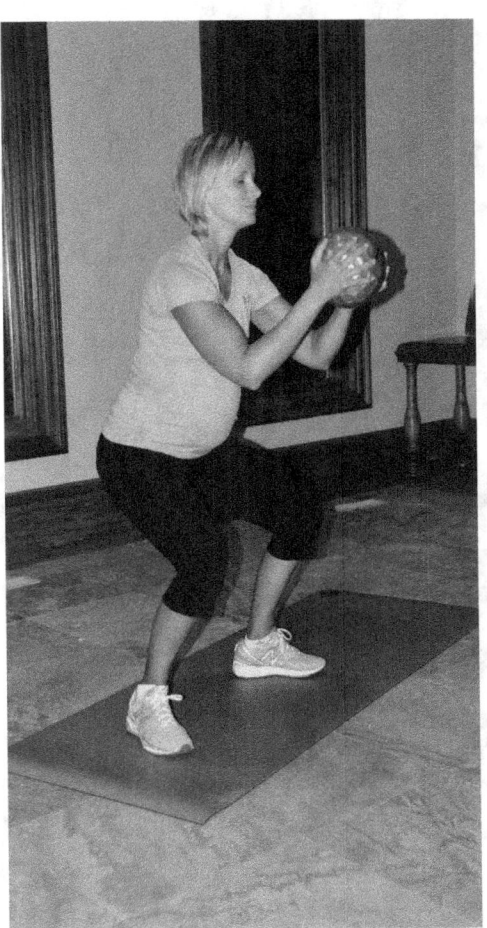

1. Start in a standing position with your feet shoulders width apart.

2. With a weight ball in your hand, bend your arms up slightly.

3. Bend at your knees until your thighs are almost parallel with the floor and hold briefly.

4. Slowly return to the starting position.

DAY 3 EXERCISE 2

Lunges

Muscle Group: Hamstrings, Calves, Quad, and Gluts

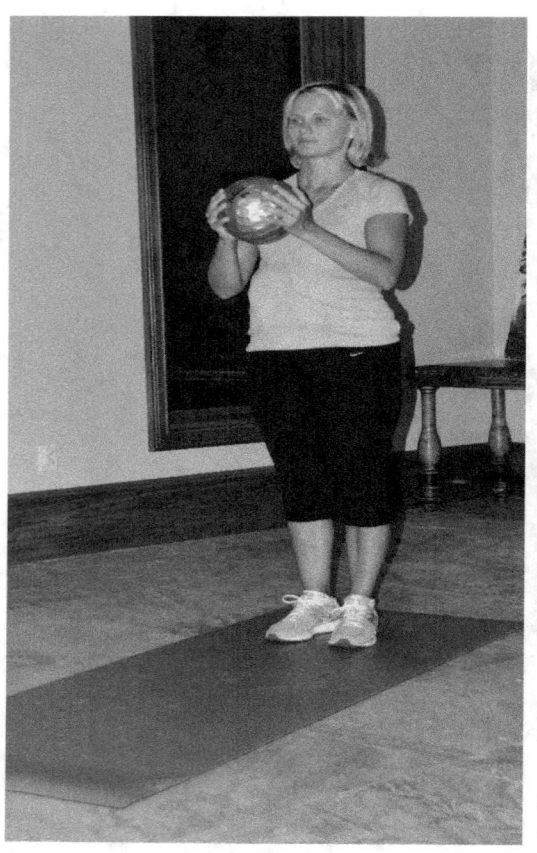 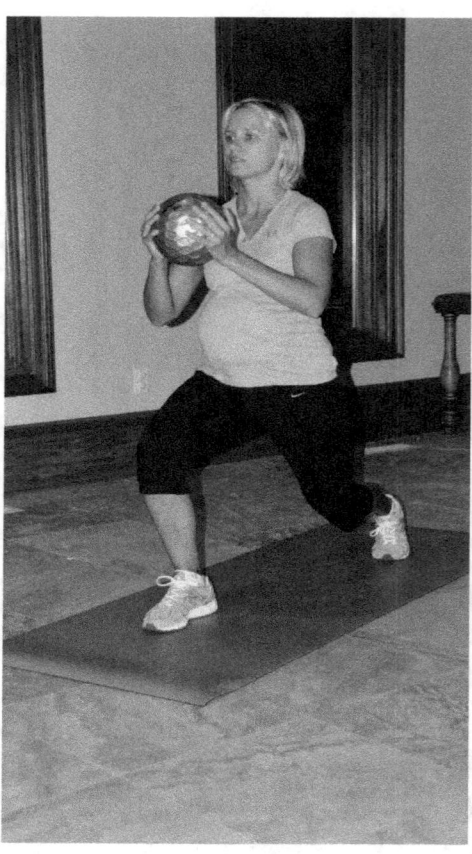

1. Start in a standing position with your feet shoulders width apart.

2. With a weight ball in your hand, bend your arms up slightly.

3. Step forward bending at your knee until your thigh is almost parallel with the floor and hold briefly.

4. Slowly return to the starting position.

5. Repeat the maneuver with the alternate leg to complete one repetition.

DAY 3 EXERCISE 3

Leg Maneuvers

Muscle Group: Hamstrings, Calves, Quad, and Gluts

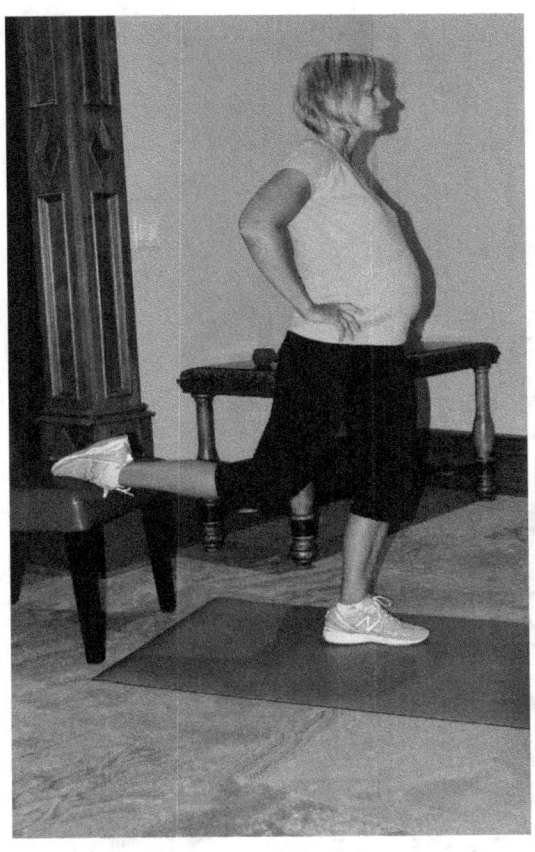 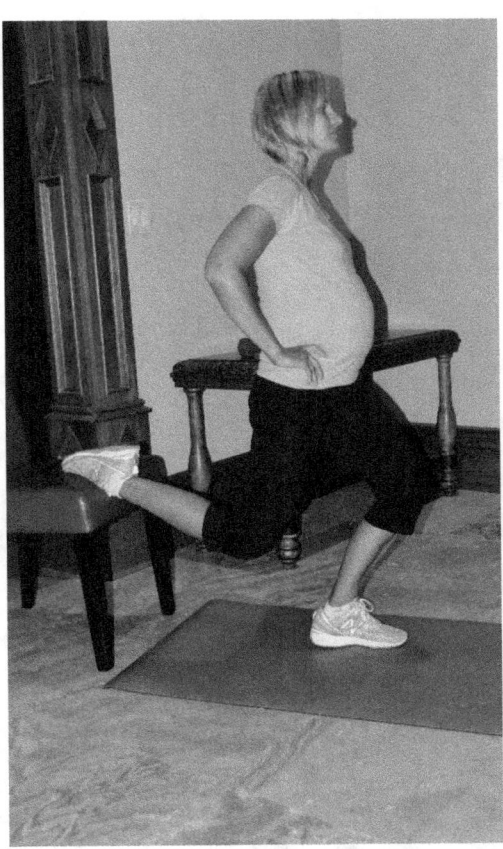

1. Start in a standing position with your feet shoulders width apart.

2. Bend one knee back and place your foot on the edge of a chair.

3. With your other leg, bend at your knee until your thigh is almost parallel with the floor and hold briefly.

4. Slowly return to the starting position.

5. Repeat the maneuver with the alternate leg to complete one repetition.

DAY 4 EXERCISE 1

SHOULDER PRESS

Muscle Group: Shoulders

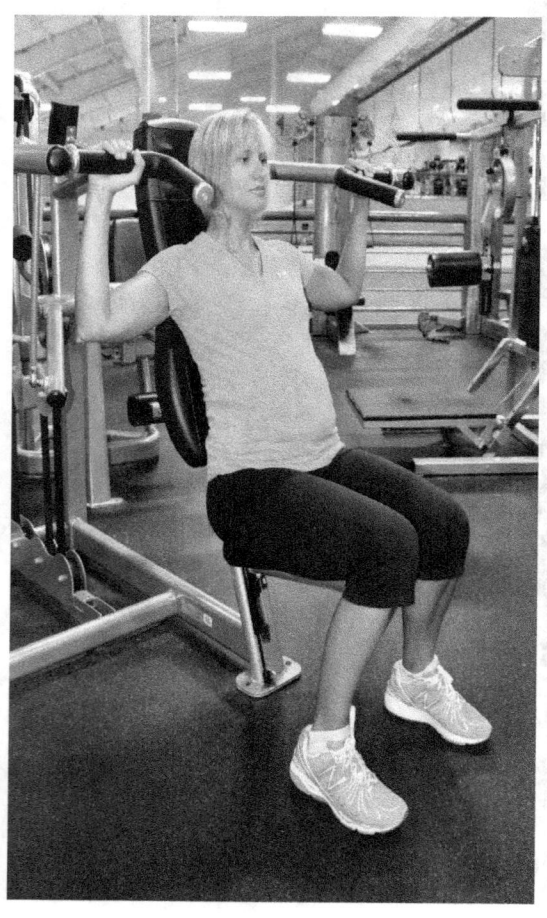 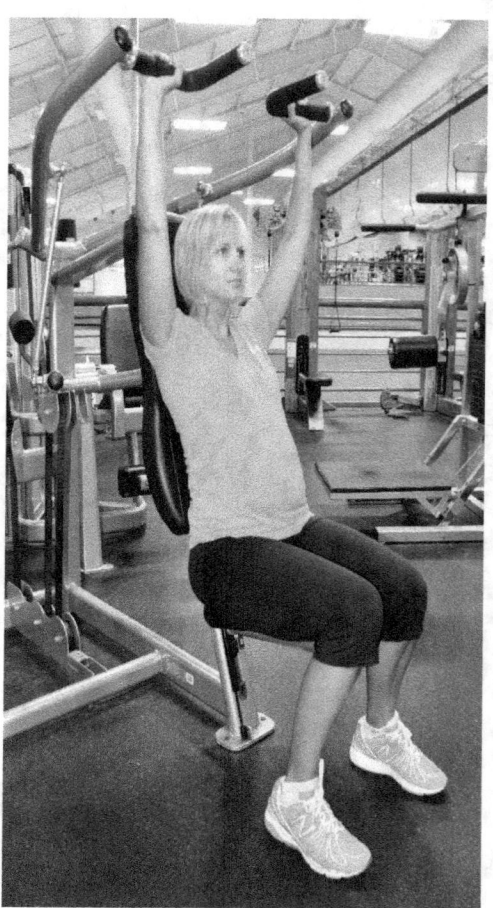

1. Grab the handles with your hands facing forward. The elbows should be bent at right angles.

2. Push up to full extension.

3. Slowly return to the starting position.

DAY 4 EXERCISE 1

ALTERNATE SHOULDER PRESS

Muscle Group: Shoulders

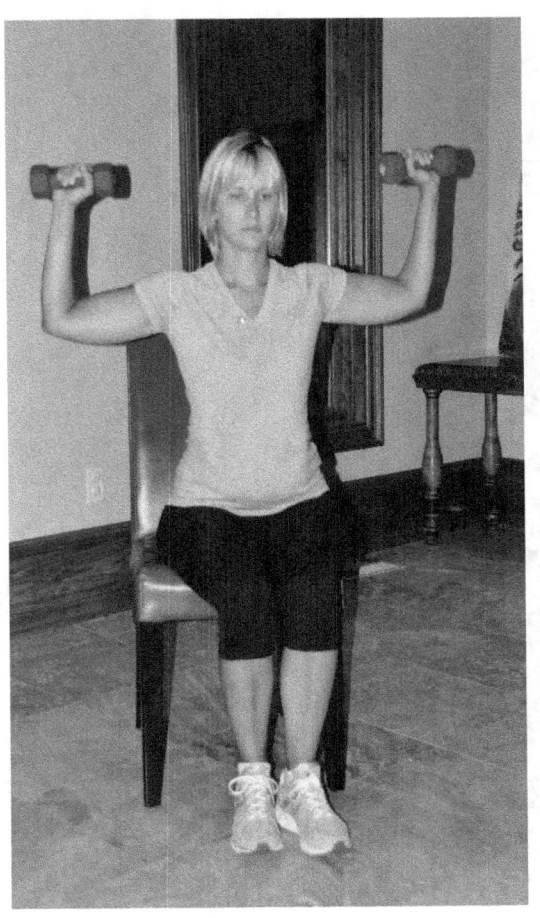 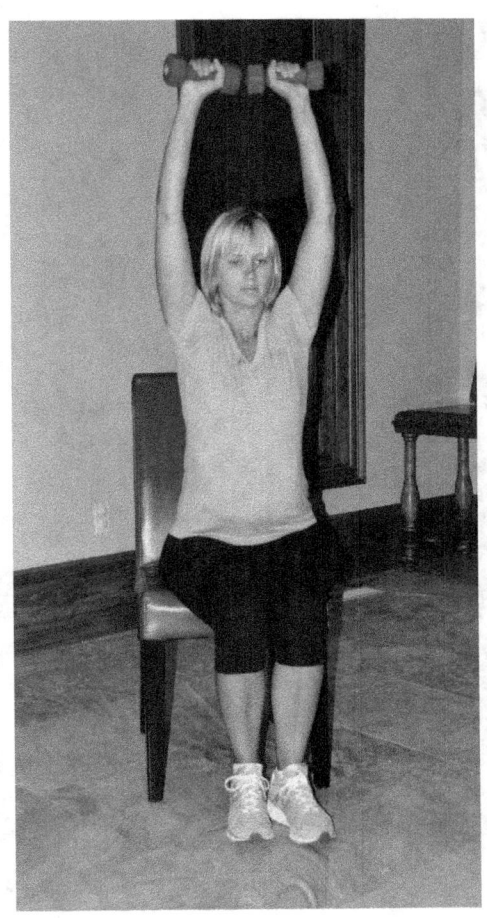

1. Grab a weight in each hand with your hands facing forward. The elbows should be bent at right angles.

2. Push up to full extension.

3. Slowly return to the starting position.

DAY 4 EXERCISE 2

SEATED LATERAL RAISE

Muscle Group: Deltoids

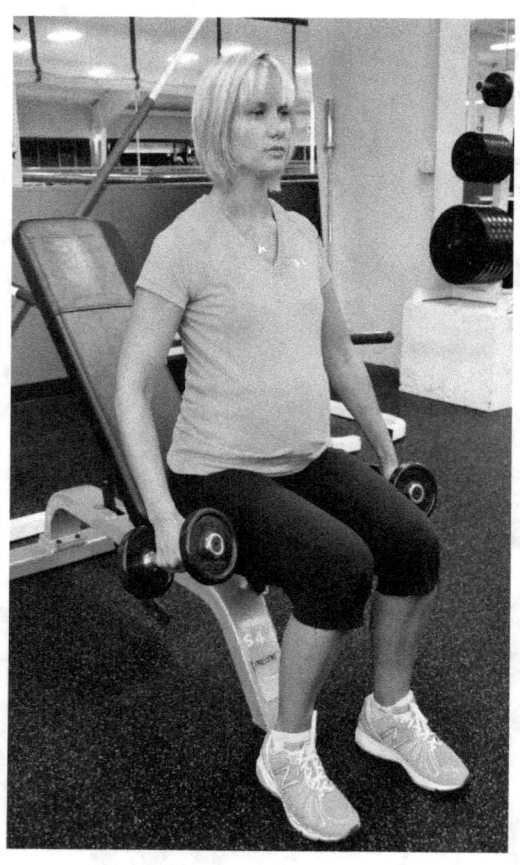 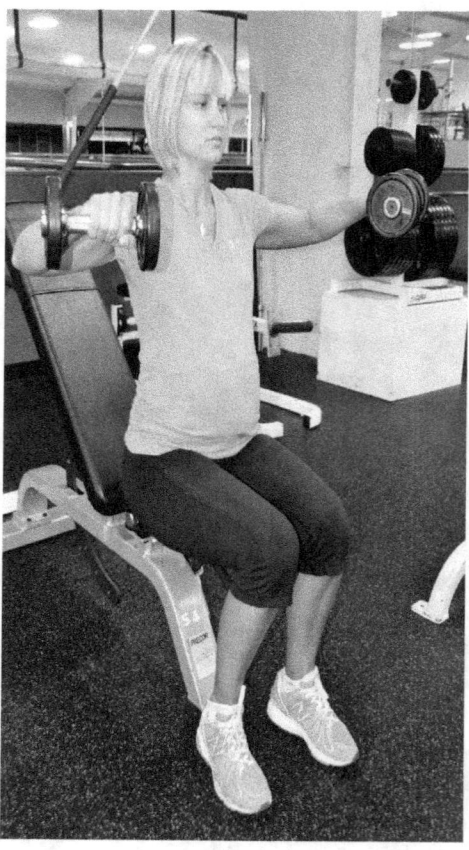

1. Grab a weight in each hand with palms facing inward. Arms to the side and slightly in front with the elbows slightly bent.

2. Lift the weights up to shoulder height, rotating from your shoulder joint. Elbows are slightly bent.

3. Slowly return to the starting position.

DAY 4 EXERCISE 3

REVERSE FLY

Muscle Group: Rear Deltoids

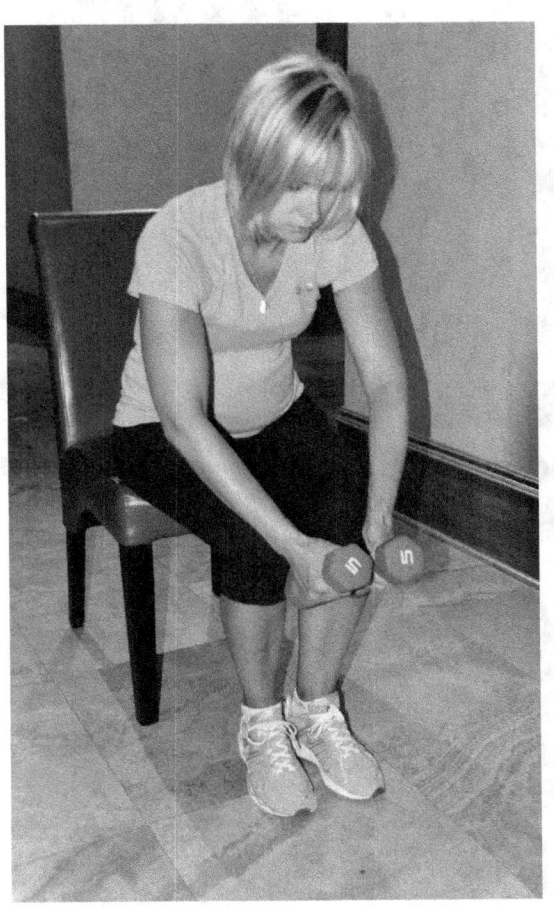 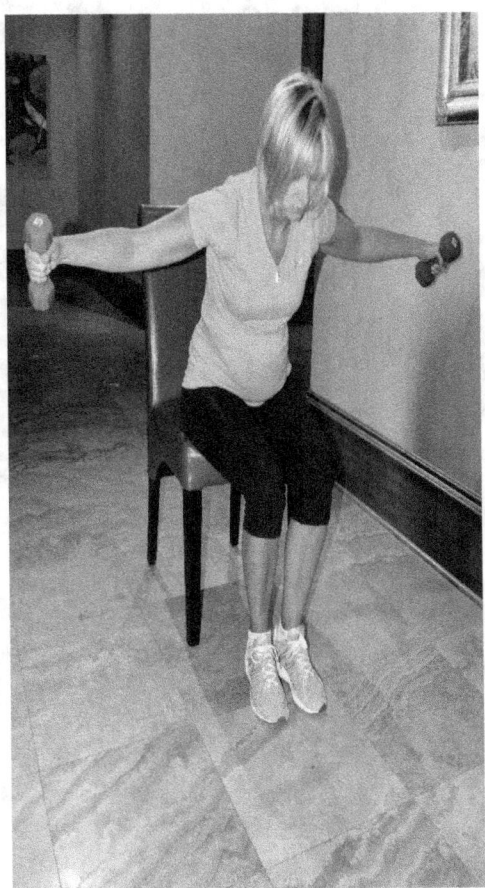

1. Grab a weight in each hand with your palms facing each other and your body bent forward slightly while keeping your back straight.

2. Lift the weights up to shoulder height keeping your arms extended.

3. Slowly return to the starting position.

DAY 4 EXERCISE 4

PLANK

Muscle Group: Abdominals

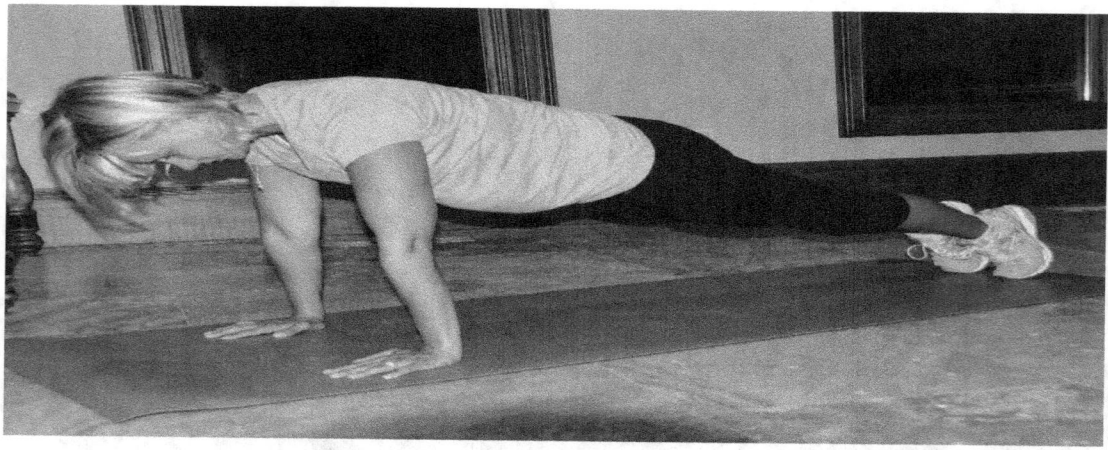

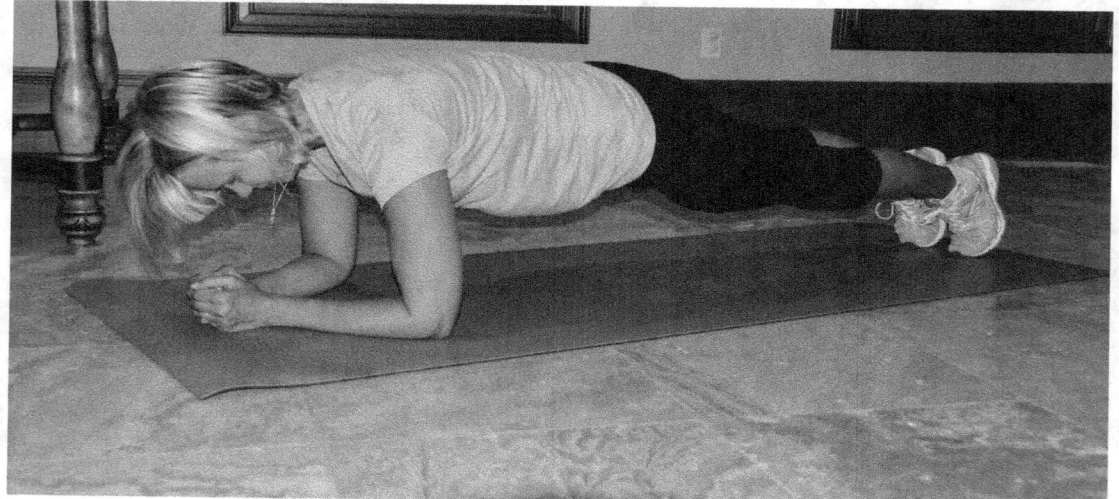

1. Get in a push up position with arms straight and shoulder width apart and hold.

2. Alternately, you can position yourself on your forearms instead of full push up and hold.

DAY 4 EXERCISE 5

SIDE PLANK

Muscle Group: Abdominals

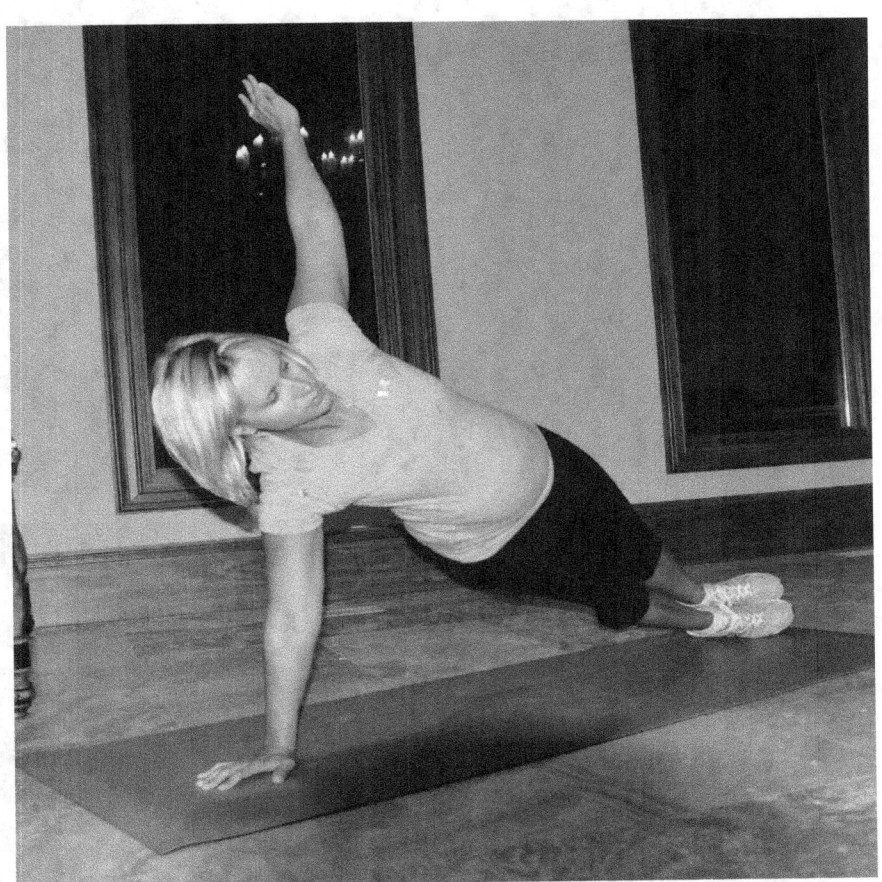

1. Position yourself on your side with your arms fully extended and hold.

DAY 4 EXERCISE 6

BIRD DOG

Muscle Group: Abdominals

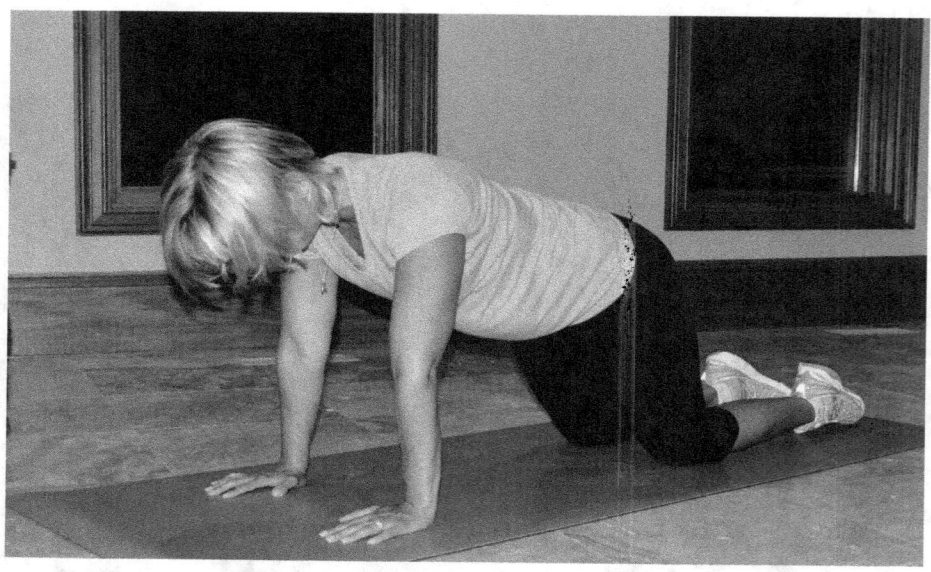

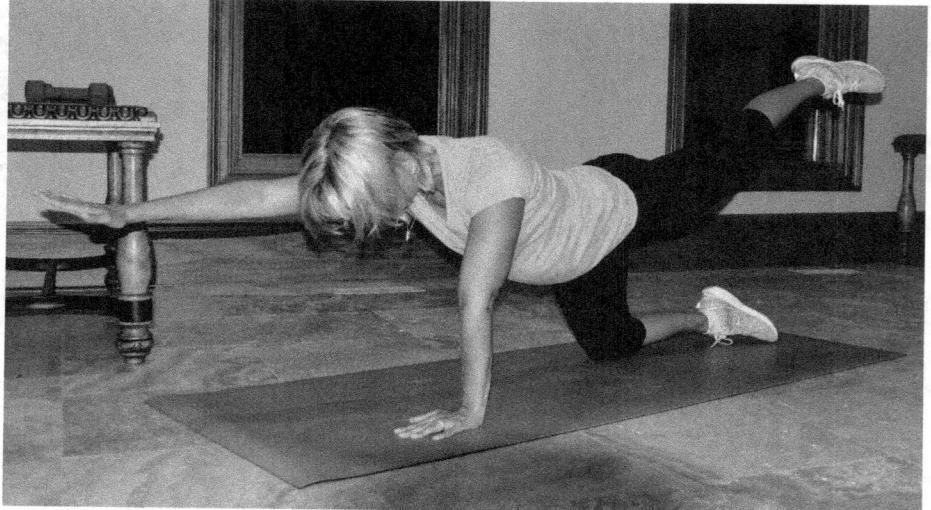

1. Position yourself on hands and knees.

2. Extend right arm straight out and at the same time extend the left leg out and hold.

3. Repeat with opposite arm and opposite leg to complete one repetition.

CYCLE 1

First Trimester

HOW TO USE THESE CHARTS

- Record your seat position for each exercise when needed.
- Record the weight of your last set in the top part of box.
- Record the number of repetitions you achieved in the last set in bottom of box.
- Start in Week 1 column.

CYCLE INSTRUCTIONS

- 2 warm up sets.
- 3 working sets.
- 5 repetitions.
- You should not be able to finish 5 repetitions on the final set without struggling. If you do, then advance weight by 5-10%.
- 3 minute rest intervals between sets.
- For abdominals do as many repetitions as you can for a set. Repeat for 3 sets. Record in the box the number of repetitions you achieved in your last set.

HOW TO PICK YOUR WEIGHT

- At the beginning of the cycle, for each exercise, start with a relatively light weight for you. If you can easily do 20 repetitions, then you know that you need to try a heavier weight. Try doubling the weight. If you drop down to 10 reps, then you need to keep increasing the weight, maybe by ¼, until you reach the point where you can do six repetitions with effort. The weight should be heavy enough that by the third set, you can only do 3-4 repetitions. When you can finish all 6 repetitions without struggling, it's time to move up. As a rule thumb, increase your working load by about 5-10% at a time.

DAY 1

Chest and Biceps

Exercise	Seat	Week 1	Week 2	Week 3	Week 4	Week 5	Week 6
Chest Press							
Incline Press							
Fly Maneuver							
Dumbbell Curl							

CYCLE 1 INSTRUCTIONS

1. 2 warm up sets (50-60% of your working load)
2. 3 working sets
3. 5 repetitions each set
4. If you finish 5 repetitions on final set without struggling then increase your weight by 5-10%
5. 3 minute of rest between sets

DAY 2

Back and Triceps

Exercise	Seat	Week 1	Week 2	Week 3	Week 4	Week 5	Week 6
Lat Pull Down							
Seated Row							
Seated Wide-Row							
Triceps Push Down							
Triceps Extension							

CYCLE 1 INSTRUCTIONS

1. 2 warm up sets (50-60% of your working load)
2. 3 working sets
3. 5 repetitions each set
4. If you finish 5 repetitions on final set without struggling then increase your weight by 5-10%
5. 3 minute of rest between sets

DAY 3

Lower Body and Legs

Exercise	Seat	Week 1	Week 2	Week 3	Week 4	Week 5	Week 6
Squat							
Lunges							
Leg Maneuver							

CYCLE 1 INSTRUCTIONS

1. 2 warm up sets (50-60% of your working load)
2. 3 working sets
3. 5 repetitions each set
4. If you finish 5 repetitions on final set without struggling then increase your weight by 5-10%
5. 3 minute of rest between sets

DAY 4

Shoulder and Abdominals

Exercise	Seat	Week 1	Week 2	Week 3	Week 4	Week 5	Week 6
Shoulder Press							
Seated Lateral Raise							
Reverse Fly							
Plank							
Side Plank							
Bird Dog							

CYCLE 1 INSTRUCTIONS

1. 2 warm up sets (50-60% of your working load)
2. 3 working sets
3. 5 repetitions each set (On abdominals do as many repetitions as you can for 3 sets)
4. If you finish 5 repetitions on final set without struggling then increase your weight by 5-10%
5. 3 minute of rest between sets

CYCLE 2

Second Trimester

HOW TO USE THESE CHARTS

- Record your seat position for each exercise when needed.
- Record the weight of your last set in the top part of box.
- Record the number of repetitions you achieved in the last set in bottom of box.
- Start in Week 1 column.

CYCLE INSTRUCTIONS

- 2 warm up sets.
- 3 working sets.
- 10 repetitions.
- You should not be able to finish 5 repetitions on the final set without struggling. If you do, then advance weight by 5-10%.
- 2 minute rest intervals between sets.
- For abdominals do as many repetitions as you can for a set. Repeat for 3 sets. Record in the box the number of repetitions you achieved in your last set.

HOW TO PICK YOUR WEIGHT

- At the beginning of the cycle, for each exercise, start with lighter weight. If you can easily do 10 repetitions, then you know that you need to try a heavier weight. Try increasing the weight, maybe by ¼, until you reach the point where you can do 10 repetitions with effort. The weight should be heavy enough that by the third set, you can only do 8-9 repetitions. When you can finish all 10 repetitions without struggling, it's time to move up. As a rule thumb, increase your working load by about 5-10% at a time.

DAY 1

Chest and Biceps

Exercise	Seat	Week 1	Week 2	Week 3	Week 4	Week 5	Week 6
Chest Press							
Incline Press							
Fly Maneuver							
Dumbbell Curl							

CYCLE 2 INSTRUCTIONS

1. 2 warm up sets (50-60% of your working load)
2. 3 working sets
3. 10 repetitions each set
4. If you finish 10 repetitions on final set without struggling then increase your weight by 5-10%
5. 2 minute of rest between sets

DAY 2

Back and Triceps

Exercise	Seat	Week 1	Week 2	Week 3	Week 4	Week 5	Week 6
Lat Pull Down							
Seated Row							
Seated Wide-Row							
Triceps Push Down							
Triceps Extension							

CYCLE 2 INSTRUCTIONS

1. 2 warm up sets (50-60% of your working load)
2. 3 working sets
3. 10 repetitions each set
4. If you finish 10 repetitions on final set without struggling then increase your weight by 5-10%
5. 2 minute of rest between sets

DAY 3

Lower Body and Legs

Exercise	Seat	Week 1	Week 2	Week 3	Week 4	Week 5	Week 6
Squat							
Lunges							
Leg Maneuver							

CYCLE 2 INSTRUCTIONS

1. 2 warm up sets (50-60% of your working load)
2. 3 working sets
3. 10 repetitions each set
4. If you finish 10 repetitions on final set without struggling then increase your weight by 5-10%
5. 2 minute of rest between sets

DAY 4

Shoulder and Abdominals

Exercise	Seat	Week 1	Week 2	Week 3	Week 4	Week 5	Week 6
Shoulder Press							
Seated Lateral Raise							
Reverse Fly							
Plank							
Side Plank							
Bird Dog							

CYCLE 2 INSTRUCTIONS

1. 2 warm up sets (50-60% of your working load)
2. 3 working sets
3. 10 repetitions each set (On abdominals do as many repetitions as you can for 3 sets)
4. If you finish 10 repetitions on final set without struggling then increase your weight by 5-10%
5. 2 minute of rest between sets

CYCLE 3

Third Trimester

HOW TO USE THESE CHARTS

- Record your seat position for each exercise when needed.
- Record the weight of your last set in the top part of box.
- Record the number of repetitions you achieved in the last set in bottom of box.
- Start in Week 1 column.

CYCLE INSTRUCTIONS

- 2 warm up sets.
- 3 working sets.
- 15 repetitions.
- You should not be able to finish 15 repetitions on the final set without struggling. If you do, then advance weight by 5-10%.
- 3 minute rest intervals between sets.
- For abdominals do as many repetitions as you can for a set. Repeat for 3 sets. Record in the box the number of repetitions you achieved in your last set.

HOW TO PICK YOUR WEIGHT

- At the beginning of the cycle, for each exercise, start with lighter weight. If you can easily do 15 repetitions, then you know that you need to try a heavier weight. Try increasing the weight, maybe by ¼, until you reach the point where you can do 15 repetitions with effort. The weight should be heavy enough that by the third set, you can only do 13-14 repetitions. When you can finish all 15 repetitions without struggling, it's time to move up. As a rule thumb, increase your working load by about 5-10% at a time.

DAY 1

Chest and Biceps

Exercise	Seat	Week 1	Week 2	Week 3	Week 4	Week 5	Week 6
Chest Press							
Incline Press							
Fly Maneuver							
Dumbbell Curl							

CYCLE 3 INSTRUCTIONS

1. 2 warm up sets (50-60% of your working load)
2. 3 working sets
3. 15 repetitions each set
4. If you finish 15 repetitions on final set without struggling then increase your weight by 5-10%
5. 1 minute of rest between sets

DAY 2

Back and Triceps

Exercise	Seat	Week 1	Week 2	Week 3	Week 4	Week 5	Week 6
Lat Pull Down							
Seated Row							
Seated Wide-Row							
Triceps Push Down							
Triceps Extension							

CYCLE 3 INSTRUCTIONS

1. 2 warm up sets (50-60% of your working load)
2. 3 working sets
3. 15 repetitions each set
4. If you finish 15 repetitions on final set without struggling then increase your weight by 5-10%
5. 1 minute of rest between sets

DAY 3

Lower Body and Legs

Exercise	Seat	Week 1	Week 2	Week 3	Week 4	Week 5	Week 6
Squat							
Lunges							
Leg Maneuver							

CYCLE 3 INSTRUCTIONS

1. 2 warm up sets (50-60% of your working load)
2. 3 working sets
3. 15 repetitions each set
4. If you finish 15 repetitions on final set without struggling then increase your weight by 5-10%
5. 1 minute of rest between sets

DAY 4

Shoulder and Abdominals

Exercise	Seat	Week 1	Week 2	Week 3	Week 4	Week 5	Week 6
Shoulder Press							
Seated Lateral Raise							
Reverse Fly							
Plank							
Side Plank							
Bird Dog							

CYCLE 3 INSTRUCTIONS

1. 2 warm up sets (50-60% of your working load)
2. 3 working sets
3. 15 repetitions each set (On abdominals do as many repetitions as you can for 3 sets)
4. If you finish 15 repetitions on final set without struggling then increase your weight by 5-10%
5. 1 minute of rest between sets

CYCLE 4

Postpartum and Recovery and Maintenance

HOW TO USE THESE CHARTS

- Record your seat position for each exercise when needed.
- Record the weight of your last set in the top part of box.
- Record the number of repetitions you achieved in the last set in bottom of box.
- Start in Week 1 column.

CYCLE INSTRUCTIONS

- 2 warm up sets.
- 3 working sets.
- 6 repetitions for six weeks then 12 repetitions for maintenance.
- You should not be able to finish 6 repetitions (12 maintenance) on the final set without struggling. If you do, then advance weight by 5-10%.
- 1 minute rest intervals between sets. (2 minute rest for maintenance)
- For abdominals do as many repetitions as you can for a set. Repeat for 3 sets. Record in the box the number of repetitions you achieved in your last set.

HOW TO PICK YOUR WEIGHT

- At the beginning of the cycle, for each exercise, start with a relatively light weight for you. If you can easily do 20 repetitions, then you know that you need to try a heavier weight. Try doubling the weight. If you drop down to 10 reps, then you need to keep increasing the weight, maybe by ¼, until you reach the point where you can do 6 repetitions (12 maintenance) with effort. The weight should be heavy enough that by the third set, you can only do 4-5 repetitions (10-11 maintenance). When you can finish all 6 repetitions (12 maintenance) without struggling, it's time to move up. As a rule thumb, increase your working load by about 5-10% at a time.

DAY 1

Chest and Biceps

Exercise	Seat	Week 1	Week 2	Week 3	Week 4	Week 5	Week 6
Chest Press							
Incline Press							
Fly Maneuver							
Dumbbell Curl							

CYCLE 4 INSTRUCTIONS

1. 2 warm up sets (50-60% of your working load)
2. 3 working sets
3. 6 repetitions each set. 12 repetitions for maintenance.
4. If you finish 6 repetitions (12 maintenance) on final set without struggling then increase your weight by 5-10%
5. 2 minute of rest between sets. 1 minute of rest between sets for maintenance.

DAY 2

Back and Triceps

Exercise	Seat	Week 1	Week 2	Week 3	Week 4	Week 5	Week 6
Lat Pull Down							
Seated Row							
Seated Wide-Row							
Triceps Push Down							
Triceps Extension							

CYCLE 4 INSTRUCTIONS

1. 2 warm up sets (50-60% of your working load)
2. 3 working sets
3. 6 repetitions each set. 12 repetitions for maintenance.
4. If you finish 6 repetitions (12 maintenance) on final set without struggling then increase your weight by 5-10%
5. 2 minute of rest between sets. 1 minute of rest between sets for maintenance.

DAY 3

Lower Body and Legs

Exercise	Seat	Week 1	Week 2	Week 3	Week 4	Week 5	Week 6
Squat							
Lunges							
Leg Maneuver							

CYCLE 4 INSTRUCTIONS

1. 2 warm up sets (50-60% of your working load)
2. 3 working sets
3. 6 repetitions each set. 12 repetitions for maintenance.
4. If you finish 6 repetitions (12 maintenance) on final set without struggling then increase your weight by 5-10%
5. 2 minute of rest between sets. 1 minute of rest between sets for maintenance.

DAY 4

Shoulder and Abdominals

Exercise	Seat	Week 1	Week 2	Week 3	Week 4	Week 5	Week 6
Shoulder Press							
Seated Lateral Raise							
Reverse Fly							
Plank							
Side Plank							
Bird Dog							

CYCLE 4 INSTRUCTIONS

1. 2 warm up sets (50-60% of your working load)
2. 3 working sets
3. 6 repetitions each set. 12 repetitions for maintenance.
4. If you finish 6 repetitions (12 maintenance) on final set without struggling then increase your weight by 5-10%
5. 2 minute of rest between sets. 1 minute of rest between sets for maintenance.

19 BIBLIOGRAPHY

Agriculture Secretary Vilsack statement on passage of the Healthy Hunger-Free Kids Act. Release 0632.10. *http://www.usda.gov/wps/portal/usda/usdahome?contentidonly=true&contentid=20 10/12/0632.xml*. Published 2010.

American Academy of Pediatrics Committee on School Health. Soft drinks in schools. *Pediatrics*. 2004;113(1, pt 1):152-154

American Academy of Pediatrics. AAP publications retired and reaffirmed. *Pediatrics*. 2009;123(5):1421-1422

"Ancel Keys—villain or hero?" Stop Trans Fats. American Beverage Association, News Release, March 25, 2004

Apovian C.M. "Sugar-sweetened soft drinks, obesity, and type 2 diabetes" *JAMA* 2004;292:978-979

Ballard KD[1], Quann EE, Kupchak BR, Volk BM, Kawiecki DM, Fernandez ML, Seip RL, Maresh CM, Kraemer WJ, Volek JS. Departments of Kinesiology, University of Connecticut, Storrs, CT 06269, USA. "Dietary carbohydrate restriction improves insulin sensitivity, blood pressure, microvascular function, and cellular adhesion markers in individuals taking statins." Nutr Res. 2013 Nov;33(11):905-12. doi: 10.1016/j.nutres.2013.07.022. Epub 2013 Sep 18.

Barker, D.J.P. (1997). "Maternal Nutrition, Fetal Nutrition, and Disease in Later Life". *Nutrition*, '13', pg. 807

Barker, D. J. P., ed. (1992). *Fetal and infant origins of adult disease.* London: British Medical Journal. ISBN 0-7279-0743-3.

Basaranoglu M[1], Basaranoglu G, Sabuncu T, Sentürk H. Department of Gastroenterology and Hepatology, Bezmialem Vakif University, Istanbul 34400, Turkey. "Fructose as a key player in the development of fatty liver disease." World J Gastroenterol. 2013 Feb 28;19(8):1166-72. doi: 10.3748/wjg.v19.i8.1166.

Bortolotti M[1], Dubuis J, Schneiter P, Tappy L. Department of Physiology, University of Lausanne, 7 rue du Bugnon, 1005 Lausanne, Switzerland. "Effects of dietary protein on lipid metabolism in high fructose fed humans." Clin Nutr. 2012 Apr;31(2):238-45. doi: 10.1016/j.clnu.2011.09.011. Epub 2011 Oct 21.

Bray GA. Pennington Biomedical Research Center, Louisiana State University, Baton Rouge, LA,

USA. "Energy and fructose from beverages sweetened with sugar or high-fructose corn syrup pose a health risk for some people." Adv Nutr. 2013 Mar 1;4(2):220-5. doi: 10.3945/an.112.002816.

Briefel RR, Crepinsek MK, Cabili C, Wilson A, Gleason PM. School food environments and practices affect dietary behaviors of US public school children. *J Am Diet Assoc.* 2009;109(2):(suppl) S91-S107

Brownstein J. "Public health leaders propose soda tax" ABCNews/Health, September 17, 2009

Chan HT, Chan YH, Yiu KH, Li SW, Tam S, Lau CP, Tse HF[1]. [1]Division of Cardiology, Department of Medicine, Queen Mary Hospital, the University of Hong Kong, Hong Kong, China. "Worsened arterial stiffness in high-risk cardiovascular patients with high habitual carbohydrate intake: a cross-sectional vascular function study." BMC Cardiovasc Disord. 2014 Feb 21;14:24. doi: 10.1186/1471-2261-14-24.

Cunningham E. "Are diets from paleolithic times relevant today?" J Acad Nutr Diet. 2012 Aug;112(8):1296. doi: 10.1016/j.jand.2012.06.019.

Daly. M.E., et al. "Dietary carbohydrate and insulin sensitivity: A review of the evidence and clinical implications." Amer F Clin Nutr 66 (1997), 1072-1085.

Eaton, S.B., Eaton, S.B. III, Konner, M.J., et al. "An evolutionary perspective enhances understanding of human nutritional requirements." Journal of Nutrition 126 (1996), 1732-1740.

Eaton, S.B., et al. "Paleolithic nutrition revisited: A twelve year retrospective on its nature and implications." European Journal of Clinical Nutrition 51 (1997), 207-216.

Egli L[1], Lecoultre V, Theytaz F, Campos V, Hodson L, Schneiter P, Mittendorfer B, Patterson BW, Fielding BA, Gerber PA, Giusti V, Berneis K, Tappy L. Department of Physiology, University of Lausanne, Lausanne, Switzerland. "Exercise prevents fructose-induced hypertriglyceridemia in healthy young subjects." Diabetes. 2013 Jul;62(7):2259-65. doi: 10.2337/db12-1651. Epub 2013 May 14.

Esterbrook J. "Schools that can soda cut obesity," *CBS News Health* April 23, 2004

Faith M.S., Dennison B.A., Edmunds L.S., Stratton H.H. "Fruit juice intake increased adiposity gain In children from low-income families: weight status by environment interaction" *Pediatrics* 118:2066-2075.

Gryson C[1], Walrand S[1], Giraudet C[1], Rousset P[1], Migné C[1], Bonhomme C[2], Le Ruyet P[2], Boirie Y[3]. [1]INRA, UMR1019, UNH, CRNH Auvergne, F-63000 Clermont-Ferrand, France; Clermont Université, Université d'Auvergne, Unité de Nutrition Humaine, BP 10448, F-63000 Clermont-Ferrand, France. [2]Lactalis, Lactalis R&D, Retiers F-35000, France. [3]INRA, UMR1019, UNH, CRNH Auvergne, F-63000 Clermont-Ferrand, France; Clermont Université, Université d'Auvergne, Unité de Nutrition Humaine, BP 10448, F-63000 Clermont-Ferrand, France; CHU Clermont-Ferrand, Clinical Nutrition Department, Clermont-Ferrand F-63003, France. "Fast proteins" with a unique essential amino acid content as an optimal nutrition in the elderly: Growing evidence." Clin Nutr. 2014 Aug;33(4):642-8. doi: 10.1016/j.clnu.2013.09.004. Epub 2013 Sep 13.

Guthrie JF, Morton JF. Food sources of added sweeteners in the diets of Americans. *J Am Diet Assoc.* 2000;100(1):43-51, quiz 49-50

Hall KS[1], Morey MC, Dutta C, Manini TM, Weltman AL, Nelson ME, Morgan AL, Senior

JG, Seyffarth C, Buchner DM. [1]1Geriatric Research, Education, and Clinical Center, Veterans Affairs Medical Center, Durham, NC; 2Claude D. Pepper Center for Aging, 3Department of Medicine, Duke University Medical Center, Durham, NC; 4National Institute on Aging, Bethesda, MD; 5University of Florida, Gainesville, FL; 6University of Virginia, Charlottesville, VA; 7Friedman School of Nutrition Science and Policy, Tufts University, Medford, MA; 8Bowling Green State University, Bowling Green, OH; 9American College of Sports Medicine, Indianapolis, IN; 10University of Illinois at Urbana-Champaign, Champaign, IL "Activity-Related Energy Expenditure in Older Adults: A Call for More Research." Med Sci Sports Exerc. 2014 Apr 7.

Hillier T.A., Pedula K.L., Schmidt B.A., Mullen J.A., Charles M., Pettitt D.J. "Childhood obesity and Metabolic imprinting: The ongoing effects of maternal hyperglycemia" *Diabetes Care* September 2007 vol. 30 no. 9 pages 2287-2292

Hochuli M[1], Aeberli I, Weiss A, Hersberger M, Troxler H, Gerber PA, Spinas GA, Berneis K. [1]Division of Endocrinology, Diabetes, and Clinical Nutrition (M.Ho., I.A., P.A.G., G.A.S., K.B.), University Hospital Zurich, 8091 Zurich, Switzerland; Division of Clinical Chemistry and Biochemistry (A.W., M.He., H.T.), University Children's Hospital Zurich, 8032 Zurich, Switzerland; Human Nutrition Laboratory (I.A.), Institute of Food, Nutrition, and Health and Competence Center for Systems Physiology and Metabolic Diseases (P.A.G., G.A.S.), ETH Zurich, 8092 Zurich, Switzerland; Zurich Center for Integrative Human Physiology (K.B.), 8057 Zurich, Switzerland. "Sugar-sweetened beverages with moderate amounts of fructose, but not sucrose, induce Fatty Acid synthesis in healthy young men: a randomized crossover study." J Clin Endocrinol Metab. 2014 Jun;99(6):2164-72. doi: 10.1210/jc.2013-3856. Epub 2014 Mar 6.

Huang T[1], Qi Q, Li Y, Hu FB, Bray GA, Sacks FM, Williamson DA, Qi L.[1] Departments of Nutrition (TH, QQ, FBH, FMS, and LQ) and Epidemiology (FBH), Harvard School of Public Health, Boston, MA; the Channing Division of Network Medicine, Department of Medicine, Brigham and Women's Hospital and Harvard Medical School, Boston, MA (YL, FBH, and LQ); and the Pennington Biomedical Research Center of the Louisiana State University System, Baton Rouge, LA "FTO genotype, dietary protein, and change in appetite: the Preventing Overweight Using Novel Dietary Strategies trial." Am J Clin Nutr. 2014 May;99(5):1126-30. doi: 10.3945/ajcn.113.082164. Epub 2014 Mar 12.

Hursel R[1], Viechtbauer W, Dulloo AG, Tremblay A, Tappy L, Rumpler W, Westerterp-Plantenga MS. Department of Human Biology, Nutrition and Toxicology Research Institute Maastricht, Maastricht University, Maastricht, The Netherlands. "The effects of catechin rich teas and caffeine on energy expenditure and fat oxidation: a meta-analysis." Obes Rev. 2011 Jul;12(7):e573-81. doi: 10.1111/j.1467-789X.2011.00862.x. Epub 2011 Mar 2.

Johansson K[1], Neovius M, Hemmingsson E. Clinical Epidemiology Unit (KJ and MN) and the Obesity Center (EH), Department of Medicine, Karolinska Institutet, Stockholm, Sweden. "Effects of anti-obesity drugs, diet, and exercise on weight-loss maintenance after a very-low-calorie diet or low-calorie diet: a systematic review and meta-analysis of randomized controlled trials." Am J Clin Nutr. 2014 Jan;99(1):14-23. doi: 10.3945/ajcn.113.070052. Epub 2013 Oct 30.

Johnston LD, O'Malley PM, Terry-McElrath YM, Freedman-Doan P, Brenner JS. *School Policies and*

Practices to Improve Health and Prevent Obesity: National Secondary School Survey Results, School Years 2006-07 and 2007-08. Ann Arbor, MI: Bridging the Gap Program, Survey Research Center, Institute for Social Research; 2011.*http://www.bridgingthegapresearch.org/_asset/984r22/SS_2011_monograph.pdf.*

Kien CL[1], Bunn JY, Stevens R, Bain J, Ikayeva O, Crain K, Koves TR, Muoio DM. [1]Departments of Pediatrics (CLK), Medicine (CLK and KC), and Medical Biostatistics (JYB), University of Vermont, Burlington, VT, and the Stedman Nutrition and Metabolism Center (RS, JB, OI, TRK, and DMM) and Departments of Medicine (TRK and DMM) and Pharmacology and Cancer Biology (DMM), Duke University, Durham, NC. "Dietary intake of palmitate and oleate has broad impact on systemic and tissue lipid profiles in humans." Am J Clin Nutr. 2014 Mar;99(3):436-45. doi: 10.3945/ajcn.113.070557. Epub 2014 Jan 15.

Lanaspa MA[1], Ishimoto T, Li N, Cicerchi C, Orlicky DJ, Ruzycki P, Rivard C, Inaba S, Roncal-Jimenez CA, Bales ES, Diggle CP, Asipu A, Petrash JM, Kosugi T, Maruyama S,Sanchez-Lozada LG, McManaman JL, Bonthron DT, Sautin YY, Johnson RJ. Division of Renal Diseases and Hypertension, University of Colorado, 12700 East 19th Avenue, Room 7015, Denver, Colorado 80045, USA. "Endogenous fructose production and metabolism in the liver contributes to the development of metabolic syndrome." Nat Commun. 2013;4:2434. doi: 10.1038/ncomms3434.

Le K.A., Ilth M., Kreis R., Faeh D., Bortolotti M., Tran C., Boesch C., and Tappy L. "Fructose overconsumptioncauses dyslipidemia and ectopic lipid deposition in healthy subjects with and without a family history of type 2 diabetes" Am J Clin Nutr. 2009 Jun;89(6):1760-5

Lim J.S., Mietus-Snyder M.L., Valente A., Schwartz J.M., and Lustig R.H. "Fructose, NAFLD, and metabolicsyndrome," Dept. of Pediatrics and Medicine, University of California, San Francisco 2009

Ludwig D.S., Peterson, K.E. and Gortmaker, S.L. "Relation between consumption of sugar-sweetened drinks and childhood obesity: a prospective, observational analysis" The Lancet Feb 17, 2001 Volume 357, Issue 9255, pp 505-508

Maternal Mortality in the United States: Report From the Maternal Mortality Collaborative. Rochat, Roger W.. MD; Koonin, Lisa M. MN, MPH; Atrash, Hani K. MD, MPH; Jewett, John F. MD; The Maternal Mortality Collaborative; Obstetrics & Gynecology: July 1988

Mehrabani HH[1], Salehpour S, Amiri Z, Farahani SJ, Meyer BJ, Tahbaz F. Faculty of Nutrition Sciences and Food Technology, National Nutrition and Food Technology Research Institute, Shahid Beheshti University of Medical Sciences, Tehran, Iran. "Beneficial effects of a high-protein, low-glycemic-load hypocaloric diet in overweight and obese women with polycystic ovary syndrome: a randomized controlled intervention study." J Am Coll Nutr. 2012 Apr;31(2):117-25.

Michas G[1], Micha R[2], Zampelas A[3]. [1]Unit of Human Nutrition, Department of Food Science and Human Nutrition, Agricultural University of Athens, Iera Odos 75, Athens 11855, Greece.[2] Unit of Human Nutrition, Department of Food Science and Human Nutrition, Agricultural University of Athens, Iera Odos 75, Athens 11855, Greece; Department of Epidemiology, Harvard School of Public Health, Boston, MA, USA. [3]Unit of Human Nutrition, Department of Food Science and Human Nutrition, Agricultural University of Athens, Iera Odos 75, Athens 11855, Greece. Electronic address: azampelas@aua.gr. "Dietary fats and cardiovascular disease: putting together the pieces of a complicated puzzle." Atherosclerosis. 2014 Jun;234(2):320-8. doi: 10.1016/j.atherosclerosis.2014.03.013. Epub 2014 Mar 27.

Mokdad, A.H., et al. "The spread of the obesity epidemic in the United States, 1991-1998." FAMA 282:16 (1999), 1519-1522.

Nestel P. Baker Heart IDI, and Diabetes Institute, Melbourne, Australia. "Trans fatty acids: are its cardiovascular risks fully appreciated?" Clin Ther. 2014 Mar 1;36(3):315-21. doi: 10.1016/j.clinthera.2014.01.020.

Neville MC, Morton J. Physiology and endocrine changes underlying human lactogenesis II. J Nutr. 2001 Nov; 131(11): 3005S-8S.

Neville MC. Anatomy and physiology of lactation. Pediatr Clin North Am. 2001 Feb; 48(1): 13-34.

Neville MC, Morton J, Umemura S. Lactogenesis. The transition from pregnancy to lactation. Pediatr Clin North Am. 2001 Feb; 48(1): 35-52.

Ouyang X., Cirillo P., Sautin Y., McCall S., Bruchette J.L., Diehl A.M. Johnson R.J., Abdelmalek M.F. "Fructose consumption as a risk factor for non-alcoholic fatty liver disease" J. Hepatol. 2008 Jun;48(6):993-9

Palmer J.R., Boggs D.A., Krishnan S., Hu F.B., Singer M., and Rosenberg L. "Sugar-sweetened beverages and incidence of type 2 diabetes mellitus in African American women" Arch Intern Med. 2008;168(14):1487-1492.

Peaker M, Wilde CJ. Feedback control of milk secretion from milk. J Mammary Gland Biol Neoplasia. 1996 Jul;1(3):307-15.

Recommended Nutrition Standards for Foods Outside of School Meal Programs: Information for School Nutrition Service Personnel. Atlanta, GA: Division of Adolescent and School Health, National Center for Chronic Disease Prevention and Health Promotion; 2009.http://www.cdc.gov/healthyyouth/nutrition/pdf/nutrition_factsheet_service.pdf.

Rietman A[1], Schwarz J[2], Blokker BA[2], Siebelink E[2], Kok FJ[2], Afman LA[2], Tomé D[3], Mensink M[2]. [1]Division of Human Nutrition, Wageningen University, Wageningen, The Netherlands [2]Division of Human Nutrition, Wageningen University, Wageningen, The Netherlands; and. [3]AgroParisTech, INRA, Joint Research Unit 914, Nutrition Physiology and Ingestive Behavior, Paris, France. "Increasing Protein Intake Modulates Lipid Metabolism in Healthy Young Men and Women Consuming a High-Fat Hypercaloric Diet." J Nutr. 2014 Jun 4. pii: jn.114.191072.

Robert H. Lustig, MD: UCSF faculty bio page, and YouTube presentation "Sugar: The bitter truth" ; and "The fructose epidemic"The Bariatrician, 2009, Volume 24, No. 1, page 10)

Satija A[1], Hu FB. [1]Department of Epidemiology, Harvard School of Public Health, 677 Huntington Avenue,Boston, MA 02115, USA. "Cardiovascular benefits of dietary fiber." Curr Atheroscler Rep. 2012 Dec;14(6):505-14. doi: 10.1007/s11883-012-0275-7.

School beverage guidelines. Alliance for a Healthier Generation website.http://www.healthiergeneration.org/companies.aspx?id=1376.

Stanhope K.L., et al. "Consuming fructose-sweetened, not glucose-sweetened, beverages increases visceral adiposity and lipids and decreases insulin sensitivity in overweight/obese humans" J Clin Invest. 2009 May 1;119(5):1322-1334

Sugar-sweetened beverages fact sheet: sports drinks. Yale Rudd Center for Food Policy and

Obesitywebsite.*http://www.yaleruddcenter.org/resources/upload/docs/what/policy/SSBtaxes/SSB_SportsDrinks _Spring2012%20.pdf.*

Taubs G. *Good Calories, Bad Calories: Challenging the Conventional Wisdom on Diet, Weight Control, and Disease,* 2007, Knopf; and Medical Grand Rounds presentation, Datmouth-Hitchcock,

Terán-García M[1], Després JP, Tremblay A, Bouchard C. Pennington Biomedical Research Center, Louisiana State University System, "Effects of cholesterol ester transfer protein (CETP) gene on adiposity in response to long-term overfeeding." Atherosclerosis. 2008 Jan;196(1):455-60. Epub 2006 Dec 28.

Trauma: The Leading Cause of Maternal Death. Fildes, John MD; Reed, Laura MD; Jones, Nancy MD; Martin, Marcel MD; Barrett, John MD; Journal of Trauma-Injury Infection & Critical Care: May 1992

U.S. Department of Health and Human Services, Administration for Children and Families, Early Childhood Learning and Knowledge Center (ECLKC) "Prevention of overweight and obesity in infants and toddlers"

US Dept of Agriculture. *Foods Sold in Competition With USDA School Meal Programs.* Washington, DC: US Dept of Agriculture; 2001

USDA unveils historic improvements to meals served in America's schools. Release 0023.12. US Dept of Agriculture

Vartanian L.R., Schwartz M.B. and Brownell K.D. "Effects of soft drink consumption on nutrition and health: A systematic review and meta-analysis" AJPH April 2007, vol 97, No. 41, pp 667-675.

Wang CC[1], Adochio RL, Leitner JW, Abeyta IM, Draznin B, Cornier MA. Research Service, Department of Veterans Affairs, Denver, Colorado, USA. "Acute effects of different diet compositions on skeletal muscle insulin signalling in obese individuals during caloric restriction." Metabolism. 2013 Apr;62(4):595-603. doi: 10.1016/j.metabol.2012.10.010. Epub 2012 Nov 20.

Wells H.F. and Buzby J. c. "Dietary assessment of major trends in U.S. food consumption, 1970-2005. USDA Economic Research Service, Economic Information Bulletin Number 33, March 2008.

"Why is the FDA unwilling to study evidence of mercury in high-fructose corn syrup?" 20 Feb 2009, *Grist*

Wrangham R "The evolution of human nutrition." Curr Biol. 2013 May 6;23(9):R354-5. doi: 10.1016/j.cub.2013.03.061.

Ye EQ[1], Chacko SA, "Greater whole-grain intake is associated with lower risk of type 2 diabetes, cardiovascular disease, and weight gain." J Nutr. 2012 Jul;142(7):1304-13. doi: 10.3945/jn.111.155325. Epub 2012 May 30.

G. Douglas Wood, MD

ABOUT THE AUTHOR

G. Douglas Wood, MD completed his specialty training at the State University of New York Upstate Medical University, Syracuse, New York. He is a private practicing obstetrician and gynecologist who has managed, and delivered more than 6,800 pregnancies in his fifteen years of practice. His practice utilizes both the traditional and concierge practice models. He is a leading advocate for nutritional health in pregnancy. He has provided intensive weight management services for obstetrical patients, including celebrity and professional athlete clients.

Dr. Wood recognizes the important work performed by medical missionaries in developing countries and recognizes the shortage of maternal care in these areas despite their efforts. In response, he has dedicated all proceeds of this book, as well as time and effort, to Women's Health Outreach, Inc. Women's Health Outreach is a 501(c)(3) nonprofit organization dedicated to furthering women's health to the medically underserved. Dr. Wood is available for consultations and public speaking. He can be reached at obnutritionalsystems@yahoo.com or on twitter @DouglasWoodMD

www.ingramcontent.com/pod-product-compliance
Lightning Source LLC
Chambersburg PA
CBHW081822280526
45789CB00007B/2303